YOUR PROSTATE CANCER
SURVIVORS' GUIDE

For Mary,
Lana and Arthur

For Paula,
Joshua and Jesse

Also by Bob Condor

Michael Jordan's 50 Greatest Games

The Carolina Panthers: The First Season of the Most Successful Expansion Team in NFL History (co-author with Joe Menzer)

Mary Lee's Natural Health and Beauty
(co-author with Mary Lee Patton)

Also by Curtis Pesmen

The Colon Cancer Survivors' Guide

How A Man Ages

What She Wants: A Man's Guide to Women

Your First Year of Marriage

When a Man Turns Forty

YOUR PROSTATE CANCER
SURVIVORS' GUIDE

Bob Condor

Curtis Pesmen

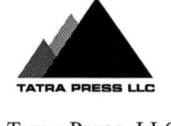

TATRA PRESS, LLC
SUFFERN, NY

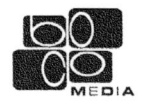

BOCO MEDIA, LLC
BOULDER, CO

Tatra Press, LLC
BoCo Media, LLC

Copyright © Bob Condor, Curtis Pesmen 2006

ISBN: 0-9776142-1-2

Designed by: Allison Ryan
Distributed by: Midpoint Trade Books
Printed and bound in the United States of America

Publishers' Contacts:
Tatra Press, LLC
292 Spook Rock Road
Suffern, NY 10901
Tel/fax: 845.357.4843
tatrapress@hotmail.com

BoCo Media, LLC
979 Utica Circle
Boulder, CO 80304
www.bocomedia.com

Publishers' Note: This book is in no way intended to substitute for doctors' care. Its publishers urge readers to contact appropriately qualified health professionals for advice on any health or lifestyle changes inspired by information herein.

Authors' Note: Certain survivors' names have been changed for privacy reasons.

CONTENTS

Introduction

WHAT'S YOUR NAME? WHAT'S YOUR NUMBER?

"We aren't numbers," said Lance Armstrong, 34, the No. 1 racer, 2-times-married father of 3, 7-time Tour de France cycling champion, and 9-year cancer survivor. And he said it loudly and clearly in spring, 2006, in a television interview on CNN about cancer and its toll, and how random and unpredictable it is. Yes, we agree: No, we aren't numbers.

And yet we live and survive by them. For the single most important change in prostate cancer diagnosis over the past 20 years has been the introduction—and refinement—of the PSA, or prostate-specific antigen test for better and for worse. It gives us a new benchmark to hold, a benchmark to guard. It's our sole, non-invasive, easily reimbursed, early-warning system (as those of us who've had more than our share of digital rectal exams [DREs] don't consider those non-invasive). For our PSA, we now know only too well, is our "Number One" Number. Is it above, or below 4.0 ng/ml (nanograms per milliliter of blood), the so-called industry standard, we want to know. We must know. And, since 2004-2005, we now know to also ask: Whatever its current level, how has our PSA changed over the past six months or year?

We live in fear of it and need to know it, but many times—millions of times throughout the U.S. each year—we need to downplay or even disregard it, at least for a little while. The reason? It's not nearly a perfect test. There are times to step back, to give doctors or our bodies enough time to heal whatever else might be causing a PSA blood test to measure (temporarily) higher than it properly should. It could be simple prostatitis (an inflammation), or maybe benign prostatic hyperplasia—BPH—that swelling of the gland with age that's normal (yet still a pain in the bladder). False PSA alarms are legendary by now, but they indeed still cause great alarm. And prostate cancer veterans know all about false alarms.

Nowadays, urologists, urologic surgeons and radiation and medical oncologists all have new options for prostate cancer patients who've already been through the Big Introduction to the disease. Welcome, survivors. This book will help you put those options in perspective.

As in: If you choose surgery, experts say the incidence of erectile dysfunction may be as low as 25 percent among men in their 40s and 50s...or it may be as high as 62 percent in men over age 70. It all depends on your tumor, your medical team and your sexual fitness before prostate cancer came along. (Most men we know would way prefer to belong to the 25 percent risk group.)

There are other scores to settle as well. Fully 10 years after an autobiographical cover story in *FORTUNE* by Intel CEO Andrew Grove helped popularize a new branch of prostate cancer treatment—radiation seeds or brachytherapy—it's time to help usher in a new era. Or three. Call it the era of combination, targeted therapy for prostate cancer. Call it the era of "minimally invasive," nerve-sparing prostate surgery; of "smarter," possibly safer, radioactive seed implants. Welcome, also, to the era of "active surveillance" as opposed to "watchful waiting."

Any way you look at it, it's time to see what else is new and valuable for survivors. Looking back, in 1996, as one of the most powerful high-tech execs in the world, Grove Knew His Prostate Numbers. But he found new ones, too, in the Partin Tables that predict tumor containment, and others that compared various treatments and their cancer-free survival rates. Plus he showed how patients can benefit by shopping for new doctors, and by becoming more involved in the gathering, and keeping, of their body's numbers.

THE OTHER KEY NUMBERS

As survivors well know (maybe too well), the risk of prostate cancer grows greatly with age. Here are the latest findings worth knowing from the experts:

AGE	RISK (of diagnosis)
45	1 in 2,500
50	1 in 476
55	1 in 120
60	1 in 43
65	1 in 21
70	1 in 13
75	1 in 9
ever	1 in 6

Another role of this book is to help put these kinds of numbers into modern perspective. Because things truly are different than they were even five years ago. Today prostate cancer docs argue about which chemotherapy to use, and when, along with hormones in advanced cases. Second opinions may in fact clash with first diagnoses. But five years ago the docs didn't argue about chemotherapy—because they didn't typically have any to use against prostate cancer.

Don't take it from us: "The perception has not caught up to the reality yet," says Tom Kirk, 57, president of Us TOO, the national prostate cancer support group based near Chicago. "Chemotherapy can be used earlier in guys with the disease—and effectively."

It is true that 230,000 men in the U.S. are diagnosed with prostate cancer annually. And it's also true that approximately 30,000 die of the disease each year. But when these two numbers are reported, it's not usually pointed out that in the U.S. today, post-2000, with better detection and treatment methods, nearly nine of ten prostate cancers (86 percent) will be diagnosed at a localized stage, when the five-year relative survival rate is 100 percent.

Now it's time, via other experts and survivors visited in this book, to go about extending that mark for 10, 20, indeed-why-not-40-plus years, of survival. Welcome to that journey. It's sure to be a stimulating ride.

As authors who have both lived with chronic illness or cancer—in our immediate families or our bodies—we won't be inclined here to hide or shelter the stark facts from readers and their families or friends. We'll tell it straight; as straight as we're able while still following the codes of balanced medical reporting. But we won't leave out the emotion. For to leave out the emotion would not allow us to be truthful, and honest, about the ugliness associated with prostate cancer. We are mostly interested, in these forthright 10 chapters, in how patients of prostate cancer in all its forms and stages learn to conquer the disease, or at least put it in its place.

"I had a guy come in whose PSA was 1,938," says Jim Kiefert, a two-time, 17-year prostate cancer survivor and support group leader in Olympia, Washington. "He was a [serious case] Gleason '9'. That was five years ago. The other day I saw him over at Costco. I said, 'How you doin', Guy?' 'Fine.' Wow. "We want to provide hope—and teach ways to cope," adds Kiefert. (You can reach Us TOO support groups at: www.ustoo.org.)

The goal of a good support group is to lend a hand, an ear, or a voice to a patient or visiting participant. The goal of this support book is to support you—and your family—in medical, social, economic and therapeutic ways. Because we think it's crucial to talk a lot more, and honestly, about what patients have found once they've entered the prostate cancer treatment community. (As in: Why don't more docs who do surgery tell their patients their penises will actually shrink during, and forever after, prostate cancer surgery? Forever...? See Chapter 1.)

The added purpose of this support book is to share information, choices, voices, and hope, under the umbrellas of medical journalism and narrative storytelling. Success is measured in large and small ways: foremost is your continued survival; and perhaps taking some new, sound health measures as you regain and reassert control over your body.

Yet success is also measured in small increments of awareness that enter the prostate cancer landscape in the years ahead: including perhaps learning about dietary support or unexpectedly weakened bladders that leak for a lot longer time than a doctor might have led you to believe. There is a lot of truth in healing, much that hasn't yet been heard. Which is what we hope you'll take home from these pages: more truth, more health, and lots more strength.

Bob Condor   Curtis Pesmen
Seattle, WA   Boulder, CO

August 2006

CHAPTER 1

4 Men, 4 Cases, 4 Survivors

Curtis Pesmen

At this age and stage of life, 48, married with two young sons, I'd rather not admit I'm afraid of a male sex organ. As a veteran medical writer, as a guy who's written a few books about the body, and as an ex-patient who fought colon cancer for a year and came out cancer-free, I've seen my share of health hardships. Yet I admit: After I rolled up my left sleeve the other day to let a lab technician pierce me with a needle and ship my blood to a lab for a PSA test— I was nervous and spoke too soon when I told a nurse I'd call in for the results in three days. Like hell I would.

The truth is, it's been three weeks and I have yet to call my doctor's office. It's fear, mostly. Not because I believe the PSA will show I have prostate cancer (I'm sure the office would have called me by now were that the case: "Mr. Pesmen, uhh, Mr. Pesmen, we'd like you to come in and re-run a couple tests...."); but because I'm afraid of whatever the number

> " It's such an attack on masculinity. The other cancers have devastating effects, but for a male to go through erectile dysfunction and the possibility of incontinence, by God, it just takes away your dignity. "
>
> —Jim Kiefert, Us TOO prostate cancer support group, Olympia, WA

is that's by now entered in my medical record. Fact is, there's now a "baseline blood." For monitoring cancer. Didn't have one when I was 38. Or 28. And whether it turns out to be 0.5 or 0.8 or 1.2 or even 2.6 ng/ml, I'll take a little comfort in knowing the "suspicious" numbers for men my age usually exceed 4.0 ng/ml. But I also know enough to know the other reason why I'm reluctant to learn My Number: It's because my seemingly healthy dad—caught unprepared—brought home a prostate cancer diagnosis a couple years ago and hasn't been the same since. He unwillingly owned a sex organ that had cancer in it. He was, we all were, afraid of what was to come....

CASE 1: HAL P.'S "NO BIGGIE"

The way it began, in 2004, it was no big deal. To Hal Pesmen, it was just a number. He had the annual digital exam, gave some blood; they ran some tests. One of them, the PSA, came back with a reading of 4.42, which was slightly high. But when you're 74 years old, as my Chicago-born and hewed father was when he got his PSA score, you tend to play it down. No biggie, just a number that's running a little funny. Probably just prostatitis, you know, minor infection of the old "semenator." Happens to all his pals in their 60s and 70s, don't we know.

The 4.42 ng/ml didn't hurt, that's for sure. Maybe my dad wanted to believe it was like the annual cholesterol warnings he'd brought home from doctors for 30 years now, except his cholesterol was in fine shape. (Plus, spikes in his cholesterol levels never sent him to the bathroom three times a night to pee.) He took care of that issue back in '01 when he smartened up his meals and went on that hotshot statin drug to lower the "fat" numbers. Lotsa numbers, it seems, looking back; none of them alarming. So after meeting with his urologist in Glenview, Illinois, Pesmen went back to his home in the leafy Chicago suburbs and took his loyal black lab for a walk.

The words "prostate cancer" came knocking, uninvited, one month later....

MY DAD, MY MOM, THEIR PROSTATE

Nobody actually said my father's 4.42 PSA (prostate-specific antigen; measured in nanograms per milliliter) meant cancer. Was too soon to say. Instead the docs figured, "We'll just watch it, for now; it's fairly normal." But as my mother, Sandy, an award-winning Chicago journalist recorded it, along with dozens of other cogent details: "Our conscientious internist, Dr. Thomas Neumann, of Evanston Northwestern Healthcare at Glenbrook Hospital in Glenview, notices Hal's score [has] climbed from its previous 1s and 2s scores to 3.74. Three months later it's 4.42. Not overly alarmed about what still is considered a low score, Dr Neumann sends us across the hall to see urologist William Cook, M.D.

"Dr. Cook [since retired] tells us he isn't alarmed by Hal's 4.42 score, either. And says: 'If I did biopsies on 100 men age 75 with that score, 96 of them would probably be cancer-free.' However, he agrees another PSA check won't hurt. One month later it's risen again, now to 4.85. [That's a 30 percent jump in four months, for those of you scoring at home.] Now we have some concerns. So when Dr. Cook suggests an ultrasound and biopsy to see if cancer is causing that PSA spike, we go along with the plan.

"Over the weekend, we don't think about it (much), while pathologists study the slides. After all, every man in Hal's family lived to more than 90, and one uncle made it to 104. They all had some prostate problems late in life, and after 85, most underwent the somewhat routine, TURP (transurethral resection of the prostate) prostate-reduction surgery, what doctors jokingly call 'Roto-Rooting.'"

But that's where the joking stopped.

WELCOME TO THE "COUNTRY" OF CANCER

"On Monday," Sandy says, "We do a double take when Hal's biopsies come in—positive for cancer. Our first reactions are shock and dismay—

followed by disbelief. Positive. For. Cancer. With a Gleason (tumor grading, from 2 though 10) score of 3 + 3, or 6, on one side, and none/no score on the other."

Officially, I find out later after talking with my parents, this score is interpreted as "average range, non-aggressive cancer," along with a "medium-range" ultrasound gauge of the entire prostate at 4.5 grams ("Mediums" and "average" ranges are preferable to "extremely larges" and "aggressives"). But at the moment my folks don't care that this score in the world of cancer may merely be "average." They're both angry, they tell me, without telling me who they're angry at. Or what; they won't say. And yet they're determined to "get this thing out before it gets us." I don't know what to tell them when they call for advice, at least not yet, but one thing I do know is: They have a solid start. Not just the numbers. Not just the cancer stage (it's early). It's the way my mother is talking about getting it out before it gets "us." They're a team more than ever, with 52 years of marriage behind them. 'Course, it's my dad's prostate gland, but somehow, already, it's "their" cancer.

"One thing we learn correctly from the get-go," my mom says, "is there is no 'one size fits all' treatment for prostate cancer. Each must be tailored to fit each patient's unique symptoms." Is she not angry any more? Or just being politically-medically correct, after she and her husband must now wend their ways through the maze, repeatedly, that is urological (if not always logical) oncology today?

CASE 2: VIRGIL S.' 'BEST OF THE WORST'

By contrast, Virgil Simons, a survivor from New Jersey who's become an innovative advocate for prostate care for African-Americans and others since his surgery in 1995, got his lousy news a generation earlier—at age 47. "Obviously, when you get the diagnosis, it's the worst day of your life," he told me. "There is no future, at first. But once you see the opportunities to regain control of your life, it changes things.

"When I realized doctors didn't have all the answers, I said, 'Okay, then, let's start looking at redefining the whole equation [of my future].' Whatever treatment I chose, it was going to have an impact on my quality of life."

Yet this doesn't mean Simons' frustration—about his cancer diagnosis so early in life—has altogether cooled. Not by a long shot. In fact he made the "best" of the worst and started a national non-profit group, The Prostate Net, to help keep men, especially African-Americans and others who may be at extra risk, "in the loop" of prostate cancer prevention and care.

After he visited a health symposium in Harlem not long ago, Simons said, "In my... 10 years as a prostate cancer survivor, I've seen major changes in the treatment of the disease: laparoscopic ['keyhole'] surgery, expansion of the types of radiation therapy and, most recently, drugs that can extend survival for those with advanced stage disease. Yet all of these advances are of little consequence if we don't find ways to better prevent disease or intervene earlier."

After I visited a prostate cancer symposium in San Francisco not long ago (which was largely about preventing disease and earlier intervention), I asked Simons if he was as impressed as I was about the possibilities presented there for future patients. "There [still] is no standard of care," he answered, choosing his words carefully as if to remind me that prostate cancer research—and funding—trails that of breast cancer by a large margin. For an advocate is not always easily impressed. "Each doctor is a creature of his training. Urologists will look for a way to cut it out of you; radiation oncologists are going to look for a way to burn it out of you; and medical oncologists will use [chemo], whatever is available." It's clear he'd feel better if there were a clear, unified standard of care in prostate cancer treatment. Experts agree with Virgil: That day's not yet here.

PSAs, THE OLD AND NEW

By the time Hal Pesmen got his Stage I, early diagnosis (see "The Stages of Prostate Cancer" sidebar, at the end of the chapter), every American man over 50 or 55 who's paid even a bit of attention to men's health had heard of the PSA test, which measures microscopic bits of protein, called antigens, that are present in abnormally high amounts in most troubled prostate glands. But relatively few people had heard of the new, "age-adjusted PSA" test. This test might have helped my dad and mom make a slightly different decision about his eventual treatment, though this is not to suggest he made the wrong decision at all. He merely thought, as his dad lived to 94 and his mom to 92, that he'd probably get a Free Pass from life-threatening diagnoses till he was 90 or so. Cancer got him instead at 74—and it hit his body and mind hard. For once you hear the words "you have cancer," you remain forever changed.

As with cholesterol tests, which are merely one measure of a few important gauges of heart and cardiovascular health (others include blood pressure, CRP (C-reactive protein) for inflammation, and VO2 max for aerobic/oxygen processing), standard PSAs aren't a perfect or all-knowing measure of prostate health (see box, end of chapter 2). They're now joined by "PSA velocity," or the rate at which its value doubles, "free PSA," which normally is used to measure prostate enlargment, but NOT cancer, and PSA "doubling time." What PSAs usually uncover is not cancer but signs of age-related swelling or benign disease—or relatively harmless, treatable infection, called prostatitis—within the prostate. This is what my dad thought—and hoped—he had.

A PSA RETHINK: THE NEW NUMBERS

When it comes to tests of prostate tissue, there are certain levels at which it makes sense to take action. Or at least repeat a test in one month as opposed to six months or a year. There's also a new "player" in town known as "PSA velocity," according to William J. Catalona, M.D., of Northwestern University medical center and medical director of the Urological Research Foundation. After completing a key study with three colleagues, reported in a July, 2004, issue of the *New England Journal of Medicine*, Dr. Catalona said: "The rate of rise in the PSA prior to a prostate cancer diagnosis of cancer... is a more powerful gauge of eventual recovery or death from prostate cancer than the actual PSA level itself."

HERE ARE THE UPDATED PSA GUIDELINES:

TRADITIONAL PSA TEST (Abridged)

Age	Value (ng/ml)	Signal
40-49	3.5 to 4.5	slightly elevated
	over 10.0	moderately/highly elevated
50-59	4.0 to 5.0	slightly elevated
	over 12	moderately/highly elevated
60-70+	4.0 to 6.0	normal
	over 12-14	moderately/highly elevated

"AGE–ADJUSTED" PSA TEST (Abridged)

Age	Value (ng/ml)	Signal
40-49	0 to 3.0	normal/healthy
	3.1 to 3.9	high normal
	over 10	moderately/highly elevated
50-59	4.0 to 5.0	normal
	over 20	moderately/highly elevated
60-70+	4.0 to 9.0	normal
	over 20	moderately/highly elevated

Sources: Urological Research Foundation, William Catalona, M.D., Northwestern University School of Medicine, Chicago; National Cancer Institutes.

CASE 3: JIM K.'S VIEW: SIZE MATTERS; PSAS DON'T ALWAYS

"Fortunately, in our groups we've had people who've had all forms of treatment: surgery, radiation, brachytherapy [radiation therapy via seed implants], even cryotherapy [freezing prostate tissue]," says Jim Kiefert, a Washington-state support group leader and 17-year survivor. Kiefert was first diagnosed with prostate cancer and had RP (radical prostatectomy) surgery—in 1989.

But beside the medical hotspots of recovery, there's one key side effect urologists don't stress, says Kiefert in a recent telephone interview. It is, no way around it that Size Matters: "Your penis shrinks after surgery... and nobody tells patients that their penis is going to be shorter!" Kiefert says. The reason? When surgeons remove the cancerous prostate, they need to cut a small section of the urethra (the urine and semen-carrying tube that runs directly within and through the prostate, and thus might contain cancerous cells) and then hitch that same tube back together and back up to the bladder.

"There's some really tricky stitchery involved," says Kiefert, who oughta' know, having had his prostate cut out at a time urological surgeons didn't know as much about penile-and-urinary nerve anatomy as they do now. "You have to pull together the remaining pieces, like using a too-short shoelace, which causes the penis skin to bunch up. That's [just] one of the issues you have to worry about.

"Back in '89," Kiefert adds, "I had the choice of external radiation or surgery. I said, 'I want that stuff out of me. Cut it out and get it out.' If you go for radiation or seeds... the cancer may be gone, but your prostate is still there. It's a choice you have to make. Well, for me, it's been almost 17 years since my diagnosis, and, to this day, my PSA still goes up and own."

So, too, does the PSA for certain patients Kiefert knows who might be best described as "off the charts." "I had a guy come in whose PSA was 1,938 [yes, nearly 2,000]," says Kiefert. "He had a [serious] Gleason score of '9,' which signaled aggressive cancer. That was five years ago. I saw him over at Costco: 'How you doin'?' I asked him. 'Fine,' he said. 'Wow,' I'm thinking... 'Some people's prostate gland leaks a lot of antigen from those cells into the blood.' I also met a man whose PSA was 6,000 and he's still around. So many of us focus on 2.1s or 2.8s. And rightfully so. But my PSA was 39 when I was diagnosed."

And Hal P., my shell-shocked father, was worried with a 4.42?

CALLING ALL DOCS; LISTEN UP, PATIENTS

Unfortunately, as my dad said early on, "They all stress they want YOU to make the decision about which treatment to take. And what in the world do YOU know about prostate cancer?" Pretty soon, he finds, he'll know a bunch.

As my mom, Sandy, recalls: "We quickly were awash with more information about prostate glands than we ever expected, or wanted to know. Anxiety builds as we consider one treatment over another. Each professional we talk with agrees: Hal is not a good candidate for surgery, a radical prostatectomy (RP), as he is over age 70 and his biopsies show his disease is minimal, non-aggressive, and grows very slowly. That's why they usually suggest the surgery for younger men with more aggressive cancer. Their bodies are more resilient. For the same reasons, they all assure us we can move slowly in making any decision at all.

"Dr. Cook, the urologist, repeatedly assures us that Hal's condition absolutely is not now life-threatening. 'The cancer is on only one side and the Gleason grade of 6 means it is the average, most common and non-aggressive, kind of prostate cancer,' he says. 'The best we can tell by your physical exam (targeted ultrasound and biopsies), is that it seems to be localized. If you were 10 years older, or impaired in any way, we certainly would consider no treatment at all.

"'Before we get too comfortable with that,' he adds, 'if you can promise you'll be hit by a car and killed in five years, you don't have to do anything.'" The bad/good news, if you could call it that, is that men in the Pesmen family have a history of living into their nineties. Some kind of treatment seems in order here.

MIDNIGHT FLUSHES; MIDNIGHT "FANTASIES"

Eliminating prostate cancer has become my dad's and mom's first priority. "We don't sleep well at night," she says. "One of us keeps getting up to use the bathroom. The other keeps waking with hallucinatory nightmares.

"On our way to meet Dr. Bloomer [of Evanston Northwestern hospital] to talk about radiation," Sandy says, "it's odd to walk through the radiation wing of treatment center, and see waiting rooms filled with elderly men, many of whom we feel sure are receiving treatment for the problem we face. Dr. Bloomer's confidence comforts us as we settle into his small examining room. To his credit, this radiologist comments that if we lived in Canada, or some other country with socialized medicine, Hal wouldn't receive any treatment at all for this diagnosis. (At least not yet.)

"But that doesn't stop him from giving us a complete pitch for radiation. He presents us with a folder filled with information and statistics concerning all forms of and all treatments for prostate cancer. In short, the feeling here is that radiation will be the best treatment. And the more we hear about daily weekday visits to a hospital for 6 to 8 weeks to undergo beam radiation, the less inclined we are to do that. Especially when Dr. Bloomer describes the side effects, which may include catheters, painful—burning urination, diarrhea, incontinence and impotence." Some party.

BRACHYTHERAPY: (RADIATION) SEEDS FOR LIFE

We're talking about killing cancer—and ridding it from the body—and the doctors, my mom and dad say, for some reason keep focusing on side effects. Unpleasant ones.

"So now we're thinking about radiation seeds," my dad says, throwing a curve into the mix. "This isn't exactly a walk in the park, either." He's just met with Thomas Keeler, M.D., another urologist at Glenbrook Hospital, who is Dr. Bloomer's team partner in seed implantation at Evanston Hospital. Dr. Keeler would take an ultrasound image of my dad's prostate and make sure the target tissue measurements are correct. Then he'd mark exactly where the seeds will be placed. Once that's determined, my dad would be prepped for implantation over a couple of hours, while remaining under general anesthetic.

A little frazzled, my mom and dad exit that meeting more convinced than ever that the seeds are the lesser of all the treatment "evils" they've learned about in this crash course to date. It's completed in one (20-minute) treatment under anesthetic, and my dad may experience fewer side effects than with external beam, as the radiation is applied directly to the cancer inside the prostate. By doing so, it shouldn't beam, by mistake, through the intestines, bladder or other organs, as it might with external beam radiation.

"The moment we returned home, we called and made an appointment for the next week with Dr. Keeler for the seed implants." my dad says. "It's amazing how quickly laymen like us," my mom chips in, "can be influenced to make a decision we are not at all qualified or prepared to make."

CASE 4: MIKE C.'S BRACHYTHERAPY SEEDS

"My dad died of prostate cancer," says Mike Carlson, 69, a chaplain of the Luther Midelfort Hospital, of Eau Claire, Wisconsin. "And he hadn't had the benefits of routine office visits and checkups like I did. His cancer metastasized; he only lived about 2 more years after he got diagnosed."

After doing his own prostate "homework" and readings, "I got the [radioactive] seeds put in 10 years ago at Mayo Clinic," Carlson, still an active skier nearing age 70, told me. This sounded sort of brave to me, as this was the mid-1990s, and the newish, low-energy X-ray seeds weren't yet widely prescribed nationwide. "But I still don't consider myself a pioneer," Mike says. "Brachytherapy seemed like the best treatment choice for me, given my age and desired outcomes. After thoroughly discussing all the options with my doctor and making a decision about which treatment modality I wanted to pursue, I was anxious to get through it."

In terms of today's modern treatments (see Chapter 3), Carlson knew the Mayo Clinic in Rochester, Minnesota, where he was headed for treatment, had a long history of first-rate prostate surgery. But he'd already settled, in his own mind, on the brachytherapy procedure. He soon learned, as many surprised patients do, that the dozen or so prostate-seed pellets (about the size of a grain of rice) aren't put in place right away. First comes an at-times tricky simulation (involving rectal ultrasound "wands"); later the seeds are precisely "delivered," or shot, through thin tubes through the perineum, between the anus and scrotum, and on into and around the prostate gland. Still, at this point in time, choosing seeds was the right decision... For Him. Another reason that swayed Carlson? "At one point," he recalls, "I said aloud to a doctor: 'I'd like to save my sex life as well,'" which at the time seemed more likely to occur with seeds—in regard to avoiding impotence—than surgery.

RADIATION VIA SEEDS, RUDY GIULIANI-STYLE

At this point, I try to help my parents a bit without "taking over" their decision about treatment. I dig up a recent *Esquire* magazine interview with ex-New York mayor Rudy Giuliani, in which he talked about fear—and his father—among other things. When he was diagnosed with prostate cancer at age 55, Giuliani ended up choosing brachytherapy, or radiation seeds, as his treatment modality.

When the World Trade towers came down on 9/11/01, Giuliani was the figurative tower left standing that day, a strong, courageous speaker, a pillar among so much fear, indecision and anger. And so I decide to send the story to my folks. It reads, in part: "'The most important lesson my dad taught me was how to manage fear'," Giuliani says. "'[In] time of emergency, you've got to become deliberately calm,'.... Become unnaturally calm. Somebody's got to be able to figure a way out of the jam. And you'll be able to do that, Giuliani senior told Giuliani junior."

HAL P.'S WATCHFUL WAITING MOMENT(S)

Okay, so my father's PSA is still high; over the "normal" border, even. Used to be 3.7. Now, hovering around 4.4 ng/ml, where it's been for three months. (It also has been held steady in part by use of nothing more powerful than anti-inflammatory, painkiller medicine.) Decision time is near. Then the phone rings: a long-awaited callback from a doc we'd contacted earlier. "Have you thought about doing nothing at all?" asks Gerald R. Chodak, M.D., a urologic surgeon at Midwest Urology Associates and professor of surgery at the University of Chicago's medical school. He's suggesting they consider "watchful waiting," an approach that focuses on regular monitoring rather than immediate treatment. My mother listens, then lets go with frustration and quiet rage after she hangs up the handset:

She thinks, "What?? Is this guy trying to kill my husband??" And then, "We've just spent two weeks listening to three other doctors describe a variety of unpleasant treatments to fix my 74-year-old husband's newly-diagnosed prostate cancer. And this guy says we should just forget about it? He must be out of his mind." But our whole family has been so shell-shocked at hearing the "C" word, especially so soon after my ordeal with Stage III colon cancer in 2001, and my sister's loss of her first husband, at age 35 in 1988, to leukemia. Resigned, we go ahead and make one more appointment for yet another opinion. He turns out to be not out of his mind at all.

Dr. Chodak is merely echoing a leading edge of prostate cancer care... one that believes, for now, doctors may be overtreating unknown numbers of prostate cancer patients. Not all prostate cancer cases are deadly; this we've long known. But doctors today still don't know which ones will be deadly. As more and more younger men start their screenings earlier in life, like me, in my 40s (as opposed to their 50s and 60s in decades past—and that was with mere digital rectal exams, before PSAs were available), it's certain that hundreds of thousands more prostate cancers will be found at earlier stages. Which is a good thing, certainly. But millions of cases, it can be said with some certainty, have or will have been "overtreated" by 2010. Meantime, my dad awaits his final decision; but truth be told, he's not a "watchful waiting" kind of guy.

PROSTATE, BREAST CANCER OVERTONES

I may be overstating an analogy, but I think it's helpful to look back at breast cancer in the 1970s and 1980s and consider: How many millions of healthy breasts were carved out in unnecessary mastectomies, because docs didn't yet know which breast cancers were most likely to recur or spread? In countless cases they did the wrong thing, even though all con-cerned thought they were doing the right thing.

"Is cure possible when cure is necessary and is cure necessary when cure is possible?" This quote, from Willet Whitmore, M.D., the "father of urologic oncology," was first uttered in the 1970s but surfaced again in 2006 at a key prostate cancer conference in San Francisco. Point being: Some patients will be undertreated and die; others will be overtreated and live with incontinence or impotence or both. This will continue, reports Mitchell Benson, M.D., of Columbia University's school of medicine, until doctors better understand how each patient's prostate cancer case differs, in both biological markers and aggressive behavior of the cancer cells. In 2006, there simply is not enough medical research to ferret out, with confidence, which of the hundreds of thousands of prostate cancers discovered each year will turn out to be deadly. And which will be manageable. For life.

CASE 1: HAL P.'S UNEXPECTED SPIKE

Six months scoot by; my parents return to Dr. Chodak's Chicago-area office for a routine PSA checkup. The doctor is in; the PSA is higher. Some 58 percent higher. It's now 7.1. Red flag. Red flags. Half a year ago, it was less than 4.5. Dr. Chodak is surprised but not alarmed. My father is alarmed. My mother is shaken but doesn't show it. Dr. Chodak calms their fears; then repeats that he doesn't want Hal over-treated. "I don't want to do something that won't help him live longer. Don't have a panic reaction to something that may be nothing."

"But we are disturbed," my mother says. "We ask again why everyone we talk to dismisses surgery—the 'best' and most complete known treatment. Dr. Chodak says it's rarely suggested for anyone 75 or older: 'No one wants to subject a person his age to all the risks of surgery when you usually get the same results for 10 to 15 years with other treatment.' He suggests we wait three months and retake the PSA. We say we can't live that way since one more jump like that may prove too late to fix it. He suggested he do blood tests again in four weeks. We repeat we're not comfortable with that. We agree to more aggressive treatment: another biopsy the following week to determine how extensive the cancer is, and to make sure the first readings six months ago were correct. 'They may have taken samples from areas that had no cancer cells,' Dr. Chodak explains. He assures us that if there is an increase in cancer cells, it still is early enough to begin treatment."

Time to decide, time to act. This time, to my dad, it's not the plain number, the 7.1, that's frightening. It's how quickly things seemingly have changed. PSA... velocity is one of the new buzzwords in urologic oncology. It's now part of my father's medical record, too. Time to decide, time to act. It's also time to determine how extensive the cancer is, and to try to verify that the first readings and biopsies six months ago all were accurate. "They may have taken samples from areas that had no cancer cells," Dr. Chodak offers. That might explain why the biopsy information from six months ago—"clean" on one lobe—doesn't jibe with today's indication of slightly more aggressive prostate cancer cell behavior. My dad is unusually quiet through most of the latest reporting.

CASE 1: HAL P.'S EXTERNAL RADIATION, PLUS HORMONES

Two days after the new biopsy, Dr. Chodak phones to report it shows a Gleason score of 3+3 on one side and 3+4 on the other. That's a 6 and a 7 on the Gleason scale, where under 6 is okay; 7 through 10 usually cause doctors to raise eyebrows. "He again reassures us this is not life-threatening," my mom says, "and he points out that it's still at Stage 1. Translation: Very treatable. But he agrees it's time to end 'watchful waiting' and take some action. We suggest seeds. Dr. Chodak shakes his head 'no' and asks us to make another appointment with Dr. Bloomer at Evanston Hospital for a new evaluation, so they can work together on Hal's treatment.

"Dr. Bloomer raises an eyebrow when he sees the new biopsy report and says, 'This changes the picture.' It also changes his view of using radiation seedse. New twist: He agrees with Dr. Chodak... that while the isotope-powered seeds destroy the targeted cells within the prostate gland, no one knows if there may be other rogue cells around the prostate's outside rim."

Following our doctors' lead, we as a family agree the optimal decision is twofold: to use cutting edge IMRT (Intensity-Modulated Radiation Therapy) for 15 minutes a day Monday through Friday for eight weeks, along with hormone treatment. My dad's docs believe this will eliminate the problem both within the prostate and around its outside rim. Hormone treatment ("female" synthetic hormones as part of the mix) is a new addition to this regimen. Previously, hormones were used primarily in terminal cases to slow the cancer's growth for a year or two when no other treatment was available. Recent studies show hormone therapy is increasingly effective when administered with radiation and continued for a total of six months. Sounds like a plan; will be a plan.

EARLY DETECTION, SIDE EFFECT PREP

"We run out to buy Immodium AD, Aleve, and special diet foods," my mom says. She and my dad have read the lit: they expect a litany of "possible" side effects. "Fortunately," she reports, "during and immediately after the IMRT treatments, Hal has no hair loss; no 'brain drain,' just fatigue." Yes fatigue, absolutely. But no more serious side effects.

At least none that we can yet see....

The STAGES of Prostate Cancer

These are the most useful stages of prostate cancer. There are other measures, to be sure, but any doctor worth his or her salt should be able (and willing) to translate a pathologist's reading into one of the stages below, for your understanding. They are typicallly combined with a "Gleason score," which runs from 2 to 10, and is a measure of tumor size, progression or aggressive nature. The higher the stage and Gleason score, the more likely the tumor(s) will advance.

Stage I: The cancer is confined to the prostate yet it can't be felt during a digital rectal exam. Usually found during another procedure, such as surgery for benign enlargement of the prostate, or through biopsy after suspicious PSA readings.

Stage II: Cancer is slightly more advanced, but still hasn't spread outside the prostate gland.

Stage III: Cancer has moved outside the prostate and may have reached the seminal vesicles. Not yet spread to lymph nodes, an important marker.

Stage IV: The cancer has traveled to nearby organs or muscles, and may have spread to lymph nodes. May also have spread, or metastasized, to other parts of the body.

Recurrent: Cancer has returned after a time in which it couldn't be detected. May recur in or near the prostate, or in many other parts of the body, including bones of the spine and pelvis.

CHAPTER 2

Family and Friends: Healing Help

Bob Condor

As a World Series champion manager and former all-star major league catcher, Joe Torre has made his share of decisions under pressure, lots of them, with countless variations and innumerable possible outcomes. His quick mind and calm demeanor—you can just see him looking placid in those TV dugout shots during a tight New York Yankees-Boston Red Sox game—didn't help him nearly as much when he faced a big league prostate cancer diagnosis back in 1999. That's by his own admission.

"I was numb," Torre recalls of the moment when his doctor called with the final biopsy result. What helped Torre the most (and happily married men won't be a bit surprised) was his wife, Ali. She stood by his side, note pad in hand.

"I don't think I've ever felt closer to Ali than I did after I was diagnosed."

— Joe Torre, manager of the New York Yankees, speaking of his wife about the day his biopsy results came in

"Ali is the one who did all the researching," says Torre. "She went on the Internet for background medical information. She bought all the books and later came up with a list of written questions we needed answered by the doctor to help us through the tough decision-making process. By the time we eventually went to see the urology specialist in St. Louis, we were extremely well-prepared for our appointment." Sort of like having an advance scouting report. For her part, Ali Torre admits to being in denial until the biopsy result. Then she realized "the two of us" would go through the steps: diagnosis, making the treatment decision, treatment, recovery from treatment and the all-important getting back to "normal" (which for Ali Torre's husband is a bit different work setting than that faced by the rest of us).

MAJOR LEAGUE SUPPORT

"We would fight the disease both on our own and as a couple," says Ali. To that end, she believes "an extensive support system" is welcome, if at all possible to engineer. "I was lucky enough to have my sisters, parents and a wonderful group of friends who were there for me when I needed to cry on someone's shoulder," she says. "Outside support from loved ones or a prostate cancer support group allows you to feel less alone [as a patient or spouse]. You can vent your feelings and zero in on what's really important." Joe Torre says every prostate cancer patient can bene-fit from the love, support and smarts of a wife or "good friend." No des-perado stuff, gentlemen.

"That person keeps you on level ground and gives you hope," offers Torre, who routinely impresses health writers, your co-author included, who called him during the baseball season and didn't expect a callback for days... and got one, oh, just an hour or two before a big game. "Otherwise, you feel saddled with the cancer diagnosis. It becomes so easy to think of your cancer as some sort of a dark hole and that there is no way out for you." While managing the Yankees to more than 1,000 victories puts Torre in elite company, he does share a common emotion with a good number of prostate patients: "I don't think I've ever felt closer to Ali than I did after I was diagnosed."

The sudden life shift from healthy guy to prostate cancer patient is a free fall of sorts for any man. The question is, Who helps you pull the ripcord and land safely into the rest of your life? It almost goes without saying that new life is likely to include its own rearranging of priorities. Prostate cancer survivors will roundly advise you to build a team of people in your world. Find good doctors, of course, but widen the circle to include your wife or partner, as well as your children, siblings, parents, other loved ones and good friends (ones in whom you can easily confide and ones who know something themselves about cancer survivorship). You might get some of the best support and wisdom from an unexpected source— and it is entirely possible that the person you expect more from gives less than anticipated.

Building personal support and reaching out to loved ones and friends might seem elementary. But studies, like one performed in 2000 at the Toronto-Sunnybrook Regional Cancer Center in Canada, have shown that most men at first prefer to avoid talking about prostate cancer with any-one other than their wives or significant others. The Toronto study evalu-ated men with an average age of 60 and wives who were 57 on average. Lead author and researcher Ross E. Gray, Ph.D., reported that those keep-to-themselves couples were motivated by a desire to maintain life as normal as possible.

Dr. Christopher J. Logothetis, a genitourinary medical oncologist at M.D. Anderson Cancer Center in Houston, says prostate cancer patients and their wives are more willing to be open these days. He credits the public stances taken by prostate cancer survivors such as baseball manager Joe Torre, for-mer New York City mayor Rudy Giuliani and editor Michael Korda, who wrote *Man to Man*. They have all served to both remove stigmas associated with the illness (particularly related to talking about impotence and incontinence) and make it clear that they got help—and then some—from wives, friends, loved ones, co-workers; you name it.

One way to consider your support system and its import is to match it with the steps you take once cancer enters your life: diagnosis, treatment, decision. Followed by: treatment, recovery, and returning to normal. The balance of this chapter tours these very steps.

BEARING THE DIAGNOSIS

When Bob Fuhr got the call from his doctor about a positive biopsy, his first thought was, "I'm too young." He was 48 when the phone rang in early February 2004. "My reactions went from shock to disbelief to denial," says Fuhr, who owns an engineering consulting business in the Seattle area. "Then I got scared. It was a flood of emotions." For his wife, Mary, an occupational therapist, she remembered the fallen look on her husband's face.

"We were both shaken," she recalls. "I had to work that night. I was so upset I accidentally locked myself out of the office. I had to crawl back in through a window." The next day, Mary went to the school where she works part-time. She struggled throughout the day, finding it hard not to cry. The vice-principal, who had recently cared for her father during a cancer diagnosis and treatment, sat her down for some reassurance. "She was great," says Mary. "She told me, 'Once you get a plan, you and Bob will be okay. The hardest part is not knowing what to do.' That was good insight, and just what I needed to hear."

A phone call informing you of cancer is typically followed by a near-future visit to the doctor. Mary took off work and skipped a scheduled hand surgery to be "pain-medication free" for Bob's appointment. For his part, Bob created a binder to organize the medical information that he knew he would be collecting. "Bob comes from a long line of engineers," says Mary. "When the going gets tough, the Fuhrs organize binders." Mary had a unique perspective on the support her husband would need and want—and that she was determined to provide—even if she was staggering, emotionally, for the first day or two after the biopsy results.

"It had only been a year since my own cancer scare," says Mary. "I had an ovarian mass removed. Bob had been a huge support to me as we visited the oncologist. I was literally shaking so badly that I could not drive to the first appointment. Bob was a positive and calming influence."

When cancer called his name, Bob stayed in denial a bit longer than his wife. "There was a moment when my surgeon [during an initial consultation] said, 'You know, face it, you've got cancer.'" he says. "That's when it fully connected for me."

Support System Tip/Diagnosis: A cancer diagnosis is almost certain to knock you and loved ones off-balance, figuratively or literally. Recognize the 'falling' feeling as part of the process; then look forways to pull yourself up, whether it be organizing a binder for medical info, going out for lunch and a long talk at a favorite restaurant, having a good cry or, hey, even screaming into a pillow can be constructive.

MAKING WISE TREATMENT/SUPPORT DECISIONS

Former Intel CEO Andy Grove meticulously researched his treatment options and reported them in a landmark first-person story for FORTUNE magazine in 1996. His personal charts comparing treatment pros and cons impressed even the doctors treating him. Yet in July 1995, Grove put down the charts and data-crunching. "I went on a week-long bike trip with my wife and some friends," he wrote in FORTUNE. "Hours of biking are good to let your mind roam and put a helpful distance between all the mind-numbing data and yourself."

The cycling vacation refreshed Grove and put him in position to make a choice about treatments. If feasible, a getaway trip is a sound strategy for most every man facing the next step of treatment. While bearing up to an intitial diagnosis might be a time for men to keep a tight circle, confiding often in only a spouse/partner and doctors, researching and making your decision about treatment is a cue for widening your support system.

John Pearce is 59-year-old Australian from Victoria. In late 2000, he was informed of a PSA reading of 7.5 and a Gleason score of 6. His urologist promoted the positives of a radical prostatectomy—based on Pearce's age and contained tumor—but encouraged his patient to investigate other treatments.

"It was an incredibly challenging experience," says Pearce. "One of the most valuable and draining stages was a weekend away with three close mates. One a mathematician, another a research scientist and the third a secondary school teacher. They in fact had done some 'homework' before our workshop weekend including a risk analysis chart and reports on their networking with colleagues." Pearce didn't make his decision for another week. He went with surgery, but says the weekend away gave him "a sense of confidence and clarity." By that point, he knew enough, felt informed enough to make a decision.

Each of us knows just how much information is too much information, even if the subject is our personal health or survival. For San Jose, California, resident Tom McMahon, 77, his "that's-enough" point came after numerous conversations with men who had tried surgery or radiation. "It seemed every one of them experienced something screwy," says McMahon, who was diagnosed in 2002. So McMahon decided on watchful waiting. Lisa Reinhart says she and husband Mike made an opposite and quick decision, opting for surgery, once Mike received an early 2006 diagnosis.

"The doctor had ordered a CT scan to determine if the cancer had been contained within the prostate [meaning no other cancer]. 'Yes!'" she wrote in a chatroom posting at www.yananow.net (for You Are Not Alone Now). "It was this glorious news, along with Mike's age and good health that helped him make his decision to remove the prostate. Get it out of his body! As soon as feasibly possible.... All family members agreed with this decision, so the surgery was scheduled. It would be laparoscopic (minimally invasive surgery), performed with the use of the newfangled daVinci machine.

"I believe Mike would have admitted himself to the hospital that day, in such a rush to get it out, but of course, there is a waiting period after the biopsies to allow things internally to settle down and heal after the biopsy intrusion and trauma."

Support System TipTreatment Decision: It pays to do your research homework, which you of course are doing in part doing by reading this book. Get second or third opinions from doctors and other medical practitioners, when possible, but try to also solicit opinions from other prostate cancer survivors, who may be more candid about results and side effects. Don't hesitate to go to reputable Internet sites for patient stories and mentoring. And, make a point to know, at the gut level, when enough information is enough for the best treatment decision. Be sure to carve out some emotional breathing room before any decision.

TALES FROM THE FRONT (PART I)

Some of the best support during your treatment can come from other men who followed your course ahead of you. Many medical centers have prostate support groups that meet for discussion and lectures. Another viable option is seeking out the cancer support organizations with local chapters and/or facilities in your area. One quick example: Metropolitan Chicago has four distinct cancer support and wellness centers devoted solely to supporting patients and families, and dozens more centers with cancer support services. These days, you can also glean a good amount of information from Internet sites such as those operated by Us TOO, You Are Not Alone Now, Male Care and many more (see Chapter 10). Men and their loved ones will likely find some of the best advice coming from guys and their wives who are candid about what worked and didn't work so well during their therapies. You can feel free to reach out to these Internet sites or call centers at any point during your treatment—even late at night when you can't sleep. There are message boards and mentor postings designed to provide both comfort and confidence to men.

Texan Danny Staggs went to his first local prostate cancer support group in March 2006, just a day after his preparation visit for brachtherapy. He attended a lecture by an Austin, Texas, urologist, Dr. Randy Fagin, who specializes in robotic, laparoscopic prosatectomies (which sound almost simpler to perform than to say aloud). Staggs was impressed enough to investigate the option and eventually decided to choose this procedure over the seeds. One persuasive point: Fagin said his patients averaged just two incontinence pads a day within six weeks of surgery and "it improves from there."

Staggs' late-March surgery went well. He wore a catheter for six days; on the day of its removal, Staggs got the "wonderful news that all margins were negative." Staggs did report one problem in his postings at the prostate cancer support site www.yananow.net:

"I had post-surgery bladder spasms. They felt as though someone was trying to electrocute me thru the tip of my penis. This, even though I was taking bladder spasm medication as part of my post-surgery drug regimen. I had to call the doctor at 10 p.m. on a Sunday night and he called in Xanax (a sedative) to my pharmacy. With the catheter, I had no need to get up at night and, with the Xanax, I slept for seven-and-a-half hours that night!"

By May, Staggs was feeling much better and walking three miles per day. He posted this checklist to help and support other men and their wives through treatment. It offers a number of valuable, "if only I knew then what I know now" items:

1. The ONLY way you can ever be sure that your prostate cancer is staged correctly is to have your prostate removed. Once it's removed it can be analyzed completely by a pathologist. Then you know whether the biopsy was correct and the treatment appropriate.

2. ALWAYS get a second opinion from another surgeon—preferably from a surgeon who does a different procedure (e.g. one 'open prostatectomy' and one laparoscopic).

3. If you have brachytherapy and it doesn't eradicate the prostate cancer, you CAN'T have additional radiation. You've eliminated radiation as a backup plan.

4. If you have radiation (including brachytherapy) and it doesn't eradicate the prostate cancer, it's highly unlikely that you will be able to have "salvage surgery." I've been told it is 'just too messy' because of the scarring caused by the radiation.

COUPLES' TREATMENT CONFESSIONS

Nobody said it'd be easy. Indeed, a recent Roper Starch Worldwide research survey of spouses showed that 83 percent of wives said they play a key role in boosting their husbands' morale during treatment. Two-thirds of the wife respondents said they accompany spouses to treatment, while 59 percent saw it as their duty to make sure their husbands follow the treatment regimen.

The tough truths? Some 42 percent of the wives reported additional stress, sleeplessness and weight swings during their husbands' treatment periods. Fully half of the women reported feelings of helplessness, loss of intimacy, anxiety and depression. Through it all, however, 41 percent of the spouses said they became closer to their men because of the disease.

THE ART OF RETURNING TO "NORMAL"

We all have a different sense of what's normal. I'm guessing my home with two bubbly, non-stop nine-year-olds has its "normal" thermostat on a different setting than the one at your place. So this whole business of getting back to normal after prostate cancer is highly personal. It does help, however, the experts say, to both picture it and then live it.

For Houston resident Leonard Wolff, that image translated to long week-ends with his wife, Dee, at their farm in Burton, Texas. Oh, and regular fishing trips at their beach house in Galveston. "My family jokes with me that if there's a glass half full of water, I'll throw a lure in it," says Wolff, who chose laparoscopic surgery at M.D. Anderson Cancer Center in part because of the prospect of his getting back to normal more quickly.

"I took a nap every day for two weeks following surgery just to get through the day," says Wolff, describing his at-home recovery period.

"However, after that I was able to do all of the things I enjoyed before my cancer diagnosis. I visit the gym daily and make it a point to spend time with those important to me."

TREATMENT: TALES FROM THE FRONT (PART II)

When Ludwick Papaurelis' mother heard her son was diagnosed with prostate cancer, she had a simple explanation. She looked Marija Papaurelis, Ludwick's wife, square in the eye and said, "It was your cooking." Marija's first reaction, honestly, was she "didn't expect to cry" at her mother-in-law's funeral.

"In any case, I felt that access to a very important support system slammed shut in my face," says Marija, who lives with her husband in Montreal, Canada. That was Marija's first big shock. The next one came during Ludwick's hormonal drug therapy. Over time her strong, reliable husband sank into a depression. "I was caught off-guard," she says. "My initial reaction when it started was to wonder: 'Is he losing it? Is it aging? Burnout?

"IS THIS THE END OF OUR MARRIAGE?"

Marija admits to becoming frustrated at times with Ludwick's behaviors and even "tuning out" to her husband, which she looks back to realize only compounded her husband's "misery." She says her "eureka! moment" came during the couple's first visit to a support group meeting in west Montreal. The group included patients and wives. "It was like visiting old family friends," she recalls.

"Members greeted us and welcomed us into comfortable surroundings. When I heard other healthy-looking cancer fighters talk about their difficulties, I began to understand Ludwick and his new problems through a different perspective. Until then, I thought he'd been mostly fishing for excuses to avoid situations and commitments."

Support System Tip/Treatment: Try to find ways to tap into the previous experiences of both patients and their wives/partners. You can learn from their mistakes, and those cancer survivors are more than happy to share them. Plus, you might well learn new and significant things about yourself and loved ones.

RECOVERY AS...OPPORTUNITY

After having his prostate removed, Bob Fuhr admits to "mostly sitting on my butt. I got plumper and out of shape," he says. "I figured I had cancer and that was the way it was going to be." Then a neighbor stepped in with that unexpected type of support that nearly everyone facing adversity can recognize from their own lives. Someone reaches out, does it without fanfare, and changes your whole outlook or maybe just one little thing that gets you. For Fuhr, the guy next door had a read a book called "Younger Next Year" by Dr. Henry S. Lodge and Chris Crowley (a New York internist and his star 70-something patient who tested more like he was 60). He coaxed Fuhr to read it too.

Light bulb on. The authors talked about the "bath of positive chemicals" that exercise brings to the brain and body, especially if you can be physically active six days a week. As a former jogger, Fuhr says he was "experienced with the runner's high." Fuhr recommitted to exercise. And he didn't have to look far for a motivator. "My mom is the perfect example of what exercise can do for you," says Fuhr, 50. "She swims two to three times per week at her retirement center. She is incredibly healthy, and just stopped hiking after years of doing that too. Her doctor pulled her aside recently and asked, 'What are you doing? Because you have the body of a 65-year-old.' Nobody believes she is in her 80s."

Fuhr used his recovery period to come back stronger than before his cancer diagnosis. He seized the opportunity of regular exercise, though not immediately after his radical prostatectomy. "I found the catheter as the most uncomfortable part," says Fuhr, looking back at the first couple of weeks after surgery. "I wanted that thing out more than anything."

Fuhr's wife, Mary, upbeat throughout her husband's recovery, concedes "it was a lot of work to clean the catheter bags" and knew her hubby was uncomfortable. Fuhr characterized his recovery as "one good day, one bad day, and then two or three good days followed by a step backward." Eventually, the good overtook the bad, they report. The incontinence mostly, finally, cleared two years after surgery. "I was just telling Mary I finally feel like normal when I urinate," explains Fuhr. "There is no more dull pain or sensation. I still have a bit of an incontinence problem but mostly when I drink too much caffeine. My doctor says the caffeine causes the inner lining of the bladder to have spasms."

Support System Tip/Recovery: There will be good and bad days. Try to visualize the entirety, as best you can, as building up to more good ones than bad.

Virtual Care

A friend, indeed. CancerCare, a New York City-based nonprofit group, is one of the first patient support sources for both patient and family care for those in need. They offer written and telephone support services (telephone education workshops), plus "live," online, doctor-led discussions, including regular sessions on "Living With Prostate Cancer."
Try www.cancercare.org, or (800) 813-HOPE

CHAPTER 3

Top Treatments Today

Bob Condor

In 1946, taking out testicles was the answer for survivors.

In February, 2006, cancer doctors and researchers gathered in San Francisco to compare notes at an annual symposium co-sponsored by the Prostate Cancer Foundation and three leading oncologists' groups. One session got right to the heart of the matter about tough treatment decisions among the options of surgery, radiation and "watchful waiting" for men with early-stage and mid-stage cancer.

The first doctor-presenter reported on a major Scandinavian study comparing the 10-year survival rates of men who opted for watchful waiting versus patients who chose surgery. In the end he explained that both choices yielded survival rates between 85 and 90 percent....

Next up was a German surgeon, all business, who made the case for radical prostatectomy. He talked of

"Over 60 years ago, Drs. Huggins & Hodges showed that prostate cancer was under the influence of testosterone, and that removal of a man's testicles could result in dramatic remissions...."

—2006 patient information booklet

49

"very low" morbidity; he also presented new and highly encouraging prob-abilities about men regaining potency, as surgical procedures become even more sophisticated, and successful, in sparing vulnerable erectile nerves.

(In 1996, radical prostatectomy was the answer, still, for survivors.)

Next up, a cancer specialist from the New York Prostate Institute, Dr. Potters, didn't hesitate to say why brachytherapy, or radiation seed therapy, was the best treatment choice for men with low-to-intermediate risk of dying from prostate cancer. He talked of state-of-the-art "dynamic dosing calculations," which can better target cancer cells and cut down on potential side effects.

Finally, an oncologist from M.D. Anderson Cancer Center in Houston argued for external beam radiation as the best treatment for those same men with low-to-intermediate risk. He covered the improved techniques for maximizing radiation to cancer cells in the prostate while limiting toxicity to the bladder and rectum, including the pioneering concept of hypofrac-tionated radiation therapy to expose a man to less overall radiation.

All good information, but there's a medical parable in here. If these docs can't agree on the one best treatment, then how can a man decide for himself? We'll help you with that answer during this chapter. Meanwhile, a hint: There is no one right answer, but nonetheless a just-right answer for you.

In 2006, there are multiple answers for survivors.

SURGERY: RADICALLY POPULAR

This treatment has time on its side. Undergoing a radical prostatectomy remains, for now, the most tried-and-proven option cancer cases confined to the prostate gland. For that reason, the procedure is still the most popular choice among men with early-to-intermediate prostate cancer. It is surgery that removes the entire prostate and nearby lymph nodes when necessary.

"In 2006, the 'open' radical prostatectomy is still the gold standard," says Dr. Judd Moul, chief of urology at the Duke University Medical School. "There's a three- to four-incision [approach] low on the body. The procedure is done in two hours. It is very well-accepted [with high survival rates]."

Plus, the time factor helps—as radical prostatectomies over decades have been refined to oftentimes avoid erectile dysfunction as a result. This is achieved by keeping intact two neurovascular nerve bundles that surround the prostate. Ten years ago, this nerve-sparing surgery—pioneered by Johns Hopkins University surgeon John Walsh—was still considered, no smiles here, cutting edge. Now the procedure is commonplace at leading cancer and medical centers, bypassing the nerves that used to be severed and that control a man's powers of erection. When successful, this is done without apparently sacrificing cancer control. It's a trickier procedure, surely, than prostatectomies of old; one that may add up to an hour to the operation, but it is well worth it to the patients—and their partners—who value sex, intimacy, and the prospects of a full recovery.

M.D. Anderson, the renowned cancer hospital and research center in Houston, reports that its surgeons today spare one or both nerves in about three of four prostatectomies. If both nerves are intact (which docs call "bilateral"), the rate of retaining potency is reported as 80 percent. If one nerve is untouched (unilateral), the potency rate is roughly 30 percent.

When you're speaking to a prospective surgeon in your or a family member's case, the key question to ask is: What percentage of your patients undergo successful nerve-sparing procedures? The best candidates for nerve-sparing have localized tumors (clear margins), a PSA level of 10 or less, a Gleason score of 6 to 7 or less and no prior use of erectile dysfunction drugs such as Viagra, Levitra or Cialis.

Radical prostatectomies are often labeled "open" by doctors to indicate the body is opened up with a incision that allows doctors to reach inside.

That incision is almost always made between the navel and the pubic bone (known as "retro pubic"). Once the prostate is removed, the surgeon will sew the urethra (the urine tube) and the bladder back together.

This last step raises the second major risk (along with potential impotence). Some men lose long-term bladder control after surgery. All patients will have a catheter inserted through the penis for two to three weeks for urine control. The concern comes when that catheter is removed. Men are then "on their own" to discover a personal bladder control level. Sometimes an adult diaper helps during a transition period; other times a man is back to normal control in short order.

Only a small percentage of men have severe incontinence after an open radical prostatectomy. Studies show up to 35 percent of patients have a bit of accidental leakage during heavy lifting, coughing and laughing. The typical man regains full bladder function within several weeks to a few months.

A key step to avoid incontinence is to perform Kegel exercises as prescribed by your doctor. Basically, this involves squeezing the same muscles you use to hold urine when you have to go but aren't quite near a restroom. Don't deem these exercises as supplementary. Research clearly shows men who perform Kegels before surgery and during recovery have faster and better results in regaining bladder control.

Bottom line: The radical prostatectomy offers a high rate of becoming cancer-free because the entire prostate is removed. Doctors also remove nearby lymph nodes, cutting off potential spread and giving the lab a chance to see if there is any trace of cancer cells. On the down side, you face the distinct potential complication of impotence and, to a lesser extent, possible incontinence beyond the first several months.

GOING RADICAL ON "RADICAL"

The "radical" part of a prostatectomy refers to the concept of removing the entire gland. You might say there are two new radical ways to perform radical prostatectomies. One is called laparoscopic radical prostatectomy (LRP) and the other is known as robotic-assisted laparoscopic surgery. Let's take a look at both procedures, which are options at most major medical centers and a growing number of hospitals in or near large population areas.

LRP: So far so good on the research about laparoscopic radical prostatectomies. The minimally invasive procedures appear to treat cancer as effectively as conventional "open" surgery with larger incisions. Laparoscopy involves looking inside the body with a special camera or scope. The laparoscope, a thin tube with a tiny camera, guides the surgeon to a picture of the prostate via a video monitor, allowing the use of special instruments to remove the prostate. An incision of less than an inch is required and made at the navel. Four other tiny incisions are made to allow miniature instruments to remove the gland. The procedure is more complicated and takes longer on the table, but there are decided benefits.

Among the upsides: You lose less blood, there is less need for pain medication, shorter hospital stay, decreased recovery time and earlier removal of the catheter. There is some evidence that LRP reduces the chance of incontinence and impotence. Best candidates are men with low-to-intermediate grade cancer who have had no previous pelvic radiation or surgery.

For Leonard Wolff, 64, the LRP procedure proved the ideal choice after consulting with his M.D. Anderson Cancer Center doctors. He spent less than two days in the hospital (compared to the standard three for open surgery) and his overall recovery was cut in half to two weeks.

"On a scale of 0 to 10, my pain after surgery was a zero," he says.

"C3-PO" SURGERY, ROBOTIC-ASSISTED

Robots now cut—or rather, robotic-assisted laparoscopic prostatectomy has arrived: Also called "da Vinci" after the brand-name robotic surgery system, this procedure is fast gaining fans among doctors and patients alike. The newest robotic system is second-generation, with minimal invasiveness and little blood loss as a key goal.

Rather than using an open radical prostatectomy's single larger incision in the lower abdomen, the da Vinci system guides surgeons to make six smaller, half-inch incisions in the lower abdomen through use of a small camera and customized surgical instruments. The mini-snaking camera provides a 10x magnification of the prostate and surrounding area, and the prostate is eased out through the small incisions. The near-bloodless surgery (pressurized gas is pumped into the abdomen to accomplish this effect) allows surgeons to see the gland and nearby critical nerve-bundles more clearly. Patients report quick recoveries and scars that are barely noticeable.

Nonetheless, the robotic system's newness makes it hard to provide any long-term outcome data. It doesn't appear to be any less expensive or to decrease risk of impotence or incontinence. There is some debate about whether patients recover faster than men with open prostatectomies and whether the new technique is over-promoted by some centers.

RADIATION NATION

It's wise to learn the ins and outs of radiation before deciding on a treatment. For many men with cancer contained to the prostate, the choice is between surgery (above) or radiation.

You might say the "ins" of radiation would feature brachytherapy, which is the procedure that places tiny seeds or radioactive pellets inside the prostate. The "outs" would be external beam radiation, in which x-rays are aimed at the prostate from outside the body in repeated sessions, up to five times per week for six to eight weeks.

Let's start with outside and work our way in. Here's the must-know information about radiation choices:

External beam: Radiation techniques have improved greatly in the last 10 years of prostate cancer treatment. These days, the preferred method of external beam radiation is called Intensity Modulated Radiation Therapy or IMRT. Its computer-planning element allows physicians to modulate the intensity of each radiation beam going to the prostate. This allows the most potent doses to reach the cancerous tissue, then back off as it moves through a healthy area.

The patient lies on a table with a special cradle to hold the hips in exact place, while the radiation machine (called a "gantry") moves around the table to deliver radiation to the gland from several angles.

"IMRT is clearly the standard of care for external beam radiation," says Dr. Eric Horwitz, an oncologist at the Fox Chase Cancer Center in Philadelphia. "It allows us to get a high dose to the right place and safely." The typical IMRT regimen is five sessions of 20 to 30 minutes each week for eight weeks. Here's another question for your potential radiologists: Do you use MRIs to help locate the prostate?

In 2005, University of Michigan Comprehensive Cancer Center researchers came up with a key finding: They discovered the combination of computed tomography (you might know it as a CT scan) and magnetic resonance imaging (MRI) used in IMRT external-beam radiation can help prevent erectile dysfunction. The results were published in the *International Journal of Radiation Oncology Biology Physics.*

CT scans are commonly used, but that technology alone doesn't provide a view of the bottom of the prostate. Doctors are left to estimate. The MRI offers a more com-plete image, which in turn shows the physicians what blood vessels to avoid hitting with radiation below the prostate.

"Because we can't see any detail of this area on CT scans, we just assume if we treat below the prostate it's no big deal," says Dr. Patrick W. McLaughlin, author of the Michigan study that followed 25 men. "But it is a big deal. There is no cancer be-low the prostate, but there are critical structures related to erectile dysfunction as well as urin sphincter function. Treating below the prostate [with radiation] may result in needless problems."

Bottom line: For patients with early-stage disease, research shows that survival outcomes are equal to the high rates for surgery patients. The rate of incontinence is very low, especially after the first two months. Chances to retain potency are between 65 and 75 percent, while the standout side effect not present in prostatectomy or seed implants is potential irritation of the rectum that can last up to a year.

For more advanced patients, external-beam radiation is often used to reduce the size of a larger tumor or slow down the growth rate of aggressive cancer. Of course, external radiation is significantly less invasive than surgery but there is a tradeoff in the necessity for some 40 trips to the clinic over 8 weeks for treatments.

Brachytherapy or seed implants: Notably, the survival rate data for brachytherapy have caught up to surgery and external beam radiation numbers. You can make a science-based case for using seed implants for contained cancer in the prostate, compared to a decade ago when the technique was considered promising but experimental.

Seed implantation is known as low-dose-rate brachytherapy. It involves an initial visit to your urologist and radiation oncologist for a planning session.

You will decide on what types of seeds to have ordered (there have long been two basic types with radioactive isotopes, Iodine-125 or Palladium-103, though a new Cesium-131 seed is now used by some specialists).

During the procedure, the patient receives anesthesia while doctors use ultrasound to guide the placement of about 100 radioactive seeds that about the size of small grains of uncooked rice. The seeds are sealed in a tiny metallic case and remain in the prostate after they release all energy and become inert.

The seeds reportedly cause no long-term effects. In fact, researchers are finding that seed implants cause fewer side effects compared to other treatments. Most men can resume normal activities after a day or two, while the procedure itself lasts, oh, maybe two hours.

What's more, some researchers are developing more sophisticated software to help doctors plot exactly where place the seeds. One new brachytherapy system from the Georgia Institute of Technology in Atlanta works to escalate seed doses at tumor "pockets" that are more aggressive and problematic.

Bottom line: Seed implants are no longer considered experimental. They are a solid choice for men with early-stage contained cancer in the prostate. Like its external-beam cousin, brachytherapy radiation poses little risk of incontinence. Dr. Erik Horwitz says both forms of radiation will lead to retained potency in "two-thirds to three-fourths" of the men who were potent before their cancer diagnosis.

One more offering from Dr. Horwitz about the choice among treatments: Be alert to the physician's expertise with the technique in question. "Always ask a lot of questions," says Dr. Horwtiz. "Find out about the doctor's experience, how long has he been doing it, what's his own track record. Get long-term [patient] results too."

SEEDS OF INTERVENTION: A PATIENT'S JOURNEY

When Tom Perry, 67, was diagnosed with early-stage prostate cancer in late 2004, he was looking at a PSA of 8.0 ng/ml and a Gleason score of 6. He was also looking hard at his choices. Perry opted for brachytherapy because "it was the least invasive and has a high rate of success."

Perry first underwent androgen deprivation therapy, taking Lupron to reduce his testosterone levels and shrink the tumor. His urologist next recommended implanting Palladium-103 seeds, followed by five weeks of external beam radiation, which the doctor said would "clean up" any cancer cells outside of the prostate, an estimated 25 percent chance in his case because of the PSA and Gleason score.

Making a wise decision to get a second opinion, Perry's new urologist discovered his tumor was about a third bigger than originally measured. Perry went on a second dose of hormonal drugs to shrink the tumor before seed therapy.

By mid-2005, Perry's doctors were still concerned about the overall size of the tumor, which was still above 50 centimeters (below that mark is ideal for implanting seeds). The recommendation: Five weeks of IMRT or external beam radiation, then the seed therapy if the tumor moved under the 50-centimeter threshold. If not, then Perry would undergo nine more weeks of IMRT and was told to "expect complications" and "possible worsening of the urinary function."

All of it, let's say, motivated Perry enough to investigate cryosurgery or a controlled freezing of the prostate (see next section). Perry went with "cryo" because it involved no radiation or radioactive seeds, didn't destroy the entire prostate and could be repeated if it didn't work (not true with brachytherapy and generally the case with external beam).

Perry says he experienced no incontinence by three weeks after the cryosurgery and felt back to normal in less than two months. By January 2006, his "libido was making a comeback" because the nerve bundles around the prostate were spared and he was off all drugs. Most importantly, his PSA was 0.3.

His openness to a new treatment to new procedures and a distinct change in course is impressive, even more when you discover Perry's screen name on a prostate cancer support site: seedman01.

FREEZE CONTROL: CRYOSURGERY'S NEW HOPE

Cryosurgery is an emerging option for men with early-stage cancer limited to the prostate. It systematically freezes the prostate gland to destroy cancer cells that can't handle the temperature drop. Along with the cells themselves, cancer growth is further slowed because surrounding connective tissue and capillaries are damaged, resulting in an inadequate blood supply to the cancer cells.

The procedure is at once inviting but too new to have long-term data; but scientists are suggesting cryosurgery survival rates for men with early-stage cancer will be a bit better than radiation therapies and bit less than radical prostatectomies. Newer technology is helping make for better placement of the cryoblation probes to freeze cancer cells and not healthy cells and tissue whenever possible. Yet there is a still a comparatively high level of incontinence among "cryo" patients. In any case, the typical cryo patient will spend the first 10 to 15 days post-procedure wearing a catheter.

WATCHFUL ABOUT WAITING

You know the drill. Most older American men die with some prostate cancer cells in their bodies. But they die of other causes, not from the slow-growth cancer. Consequently, a good number of urologists still recommend "watchful waiting" for men who are 70 and older. The concept is these patients have a life expectancy of about 10 to 15 years, and the prostate tumor itself is unlikely to cause significant medical problems during that span.

One difference: More practitioners prefer to describe the not-yet-treatment choice as "active surveillance," to indicate that doctors will indeed be watchful and patients perhaps quite active in complying. You can expect regular digital rectal exams and blood tests to discover PSA levels. Those tests are typically performed at six-month intervals, along with a yearly biopsy. Doctors are becoming more savvy about how to gauge PSA results, including proportional changes that are compared with the absolute number.

The best candidates for active surveillance often are men with life expectancy of 10 years or less based on age or health status. It might be an option for men with unstable heart disease, chronic high blood pressure issues or poorly controlled diabetes, all conditions that could sensibly be first treated before prostate therapy. Some men under 70 choose active surveillance if they are deemed to have slow-growth tumors, low Gleason scores or low or slow-to-change PSA levels.

HORMONE ADVANCES: NOW FOR BOTH EARLY AND COMPLEX CASES

A good deal of this chapter's discussion has focused on men with early-stage cancer and/or cancer confined to the prostate. This section considers the situation of men whose cancer has spread outside of the prostate. While hormonal drugs are frequently used for early-stage patients to shrink a tumor before surgery or radiation, men with more advanced cases (outside the prostate capsule) use the hormonal drugs to both reduce tumor size and to stave off potential symptoms associated with cancer's spread, including pain.

Other drugs might be employed for men with advanced cases, typically because tumors eventually become resistant to medications and grow despite the therapy. If cancer spreads, it can destroy the bones. So some men will take bone-health drugs with zoledronic acid to slow down bone loss and deterioration.

Other possible options for men with hormone-resistant tumors are some new forms of chemotherapy (see CHART end of chapter.). Limited studies indicate that a chemo regimen can prolong lives, reduce bone-related pain and enhanced perceived quality of life. Other research shows some chemotherapy regimens decrease symptoms but don't increase life expectancy.

Men with advanced cases might benefit from high-dose-rate brachytherapy, in which temporary radioactive material (Iridium-192) is delivered to the prostate by needles inserted through the lower abdomen. The needles are inserted and maintained for a two-hour procedure (patients undergo general anesthesia), then the whole procedure is repeated two weeks later. The treatment is paired with external beam radiation. It is recommended for men with tumor involvement greater than half the prostate or outside the prostate, or for men with PSAs greater than 10 and Gleason scores equal to 7 or more.

TOP TREATMENTS TODAY

The charts on the following pages describe the most common prostate cancer treatments currently used in the United States, including surgery, radiation and hormonal therapy.

Note: Hormone therapy drugs are used for several situations, such as first-line therapy for men not able to have surgery or radiation. Other options include pre-treatment shrinking of a tumor, additional treatment for men in high-risk groups and/or after surgery or radiation if cancer recurs.

COMMON TREATMENTS
IN THE U.S.

Treatment Type	How it Works	Best Candidates	Downside	Comments
SURGERY Radical prostatectomy	Remove prostate with incision in lower abdomen or perineum between scrotum and anus. Bladder then reconnected to urethra.	Healthy men under 70, cancer contained in the gland capsule.	Possible impotence and/or incontinence. Be sure to find out doctor's definitions.	Still considered gold standard for best long-term survival. Fairly long recovery arc, includes catheter.
SURGERY Laparoscopic radical prostatectomy	Smaller incision because docs use fiber-optic scopes to guide removal. Other option is robotic-assisted.	Men who need shorter recovery and lifting sooner; access to experienced LRP docs.	LRP new, needs more research to compare to conventional radical surgery. Not all docs experienced with it.	Theory is fiber-optics or robotics allows more precision, clearer view to spare nerve bundles.
RADIATION External Beam	Radiation directed at ab for 5-10 minutes for 4-5 days over 8 weeks. New IMRT reduces normal cell damage.	More advanced cases at Gleason 4+3, PSA over 10, multiple core biopsies. Combines with hormonal therapy.	Choosing radiation over prostatectomy eliminates potential for surgery later. Possible diarrhea, urinary urgency, incontinence.	Ask doc about delayed Impotence issues. Ex-Beam optimal for men with cancer spread beyond prostate.
RADIATION Internal radiation or brachytherapy	Radioactive seeds implanted into prostate guided by ultrasound. Lasts 1-2 hours under anesthesia. Outpatient or next day.	Men with normal digital exam, PSA under 10, Gleason 6 or 7, few positive core biopsies.	Scarring of prostate eliminates surgery as future option.	Fewer side effects than Surgery/ex-beam, especially urinary. Solid survival stats for contained to prostate. New tech for seed placement.

HORMONE DRUG THERAPY FOR
PROSTATE CANCER: MOST COMMON MEDICATIONS

Drug Type	Brand Names (Maker)	How it Works	Comments
Luteinizing hormone or LHRH analogs	Lupron Depot (TAP) Zoladex (AstraZeneca) Synarel (Pfizer)	Simulates excessive luteinizing hormone, leads pituitary gland to lower testosterone.	Analogs similar to testes removal. Injected 1-12 months. Shrinks tumors. Can cause hot flashes, bone loss, weight gain.
LHRH antagonists	Plenaxis (Praecis/Amgen)	Newer drug stops bone pain as offsets LRHR drugs: initial surge in testosterone levels.	Used in advanced cases, But maker voluntarily halted sales in mid-2006 due to dangerous side effects deemed by FDA.
Anti-androgens	Casodex (AstraZeneca) Nilandron (Aventis) Eulexin (Schering)	These drugs block testosterone and related dihydrotestosterone binding to receptors.	Fewer side effects than other hormonal therapies. Can team with LHRH analogs.
Other androgen suppressants	Proscar (Merck) Avodart (GlaxoSmithKline) Nizoral (Janssen-Cilag)	Proscar and Avodart Decrease conversion of testosterone to dihydro- testosterone. Nizoral shuts down testosterone from adrenal glands.	Some research supports cancer-prevent effect of Proscar and Avodart, Commonly used for enlarged benign prostate. Nizoral prescribed in late-stage cases.

YOUNGER MAN'S CANCER

Conventional prostate cancer wisdom once held that a radical prostatectomy was the smart choice for men in their 50s or younger. That's because their life expectancies were long and eliminating cancer is best guaranteed when the prostate is removed in an early state of cell development.

But new research performed at Fox Chase Cancer Center in Philadelphia suggests that external beam radiation can be just as effective in achieving long-term survival in men 55 and younger. The study appeared in the June 15, 2006 issue of the journal *Cancer*. It showed men in the youngest group experienced a survival rate of 94 percent compared to 95 percent for men 60 to 69 and 87 percent for a group of men 70 and older.

Researchers did make a point of cautioning that more studies were needed and, especially, that the results "don't say anything about younger patients with more aggressive forms of cancer."

One positive note for younger men who opt for surgery: Recent research shows men under 50 who opt for a radical prostatectomy are significantly more likely to retain sexual function compared to males 70 and older with the same-stage disease.

CHAPTER 4

Food and Fitness, For Life

Bob Condor

Guys do change. One behavior dietitian Natalie Ledesma notices, over and over, in her nutrition practice at the University of California San Francisco's (UCSF) Comprehensive Cancer Center, is how "prostate cancer guys are willing to make changes in their diets." Suggest five changes? Check. Suggest 10?! "They make them," she says.

"Nutrition gives you a sense of empowerment as a survivor," adds Ledesma. "Guys facing prostate cancer treatments generally still feel well, and though I can't speak from the male perspective, the fears of impotence and incontinence seem to motivate the eating changes."

Good thing. Because it is no stretch that food—while obviously not as powerful as radiation—is a new prostate cancer medicine and not just sort-of-a-good idea.

> "The point is, you can change your odds at lunch..."
>
> —Prostate survivors' proverb

Researchers are now finding clear (if not quite cure) connections with certain foods and their ability to discourage and even slow prostate tumor growth.

The same positive vibes apply to exercise and staying fit. Scientists have turned up hard evidence that regular physical activity can reduce the inevitable fatigue associated with hormonal drugs, chemotherapy and radiation. Plus, no small thing, exercise can keep your spirits up and your fat percentage down. It fairly feeds longevity.

Before moving into the best food and fitness strategies, though, there's an important distinction to make. A lot of the research associated with nutrition and prostate cancer focuses on whether specific diets and foods will protect against developing the cancer. Some studies have looked more closely at foods and eating plans while in recovery from the disease. We'll concentrate here on how food impacts your survival once you have received a cancer diagnosis. To this end, naturopathic physician Davis W. Lamson and his colleagues at Bastyr University in Seattle, the nation's leading natural medical school, presented a number of research papers in 2006 making a case for preventive foods being valuable for survivors.

"We used to think food was more about prevention than once you are diagnosed," says Lamson. "We are out to show that is not the case anymore. It appears from our research analysis that protective foods are good for prostate cancer patients too."

LOW-CARB: HITS AND MYTHS

Sorry, guys, but all those magazine stories about miraculous weight loss while downing four eggs and a rasher of bacon for a high-protein, low-carb breakfast? Not a good plan for the prostate. Studies ranging from Harvard to Greece to China all point to saturated fat in meat, dairy and processed foods as a major culprit in prostate tumor development among men. Men in those countries with diets in which meat is more a condiment than main dish experience significantly lower rates of prostate diagnoses.

What's more, a landmark study by UCLA researcher Dr. William Aronson shows feeding a diet high in saturated fat to mice speeds the growth of tumors, compared to mice who are fed a diet high in unsaturated fats. Along with cutting down on red meat and dairy products (stick to nonfat varieties in small amounts), there are other foods to limit in your diet. On a practical note, Natalie Ledesma at UCSF instructs men away from "too much barbecue," and advises "little or no fast-food stops if that is a habit."

Dr. Glenn J. Bubley, an associate professor at Harvard Medical School, says the healthy prostate diet should eliminate "bad fats." His list includes red meat, duck, chicken skin, palm oil and coconut oil (look at labels to spot those last two), vegetable cooking oils (corn, sunflower, safflower), mayonnaise, margarine, non-dairy creamers, lard (a staple at lots of Mexican restaurants, ask if it is used), cakes, doughnuts, cookies and other processed snack foods.

A SURVIVOR'S LEAN PROTEIN LEANINGS

"I believe that diet can contribute much to slowing or preventing the growth of prostate cancer," says Lawrence Bookbinder, a 70-something Californian, survivor since 2000, and a mentor at the You Are Not Alone Now website (www.yananow.net). "I continue to avoid beef, lamb, pork, bacon, ham, duck, goose, dark-meat chicken, dark-meat turkey, egg yolks, cheese, butter and whole milk. I continue to eat breast of turkey, breast of chicken, and fish."

Bookbinder says he tries to limit his animal protein servings to one per day, including no more than one cup of yogurt or nonfat milk. In his mind, it has helped to keep his PSA level in a stagnant state for six years while avoiding any treatment except a low dose of the hormone-inhibiting drug Avodart.

"I believe I would be healthier if all of my protein came from plants, but I do have to be flexible," he explains. "I obtain much of my protein from soy, tofu, nuts, legumes, whole grain and seeds. I have soy in some form every day."

Bookbinder has made the adjustment from his once-staple white-flour foods and gained a new appreciation for the heartier flavor of whole grains: "I prefer whole grains; for example, brown instead of white rice, 100 percent whole wheat bread instead of partial whole wheat bread or white bread. The better alternative is a diet rich in plant foods, including fruits, veggies, whole grains, beans and legumes (lentils, garbanzos)."

PROSTATE POWERHOUSE FOODS: (PART I)

(ONE TOMATO, TWO...)
Full disclosure here: There is no one diet that unequivocally prevents prostate cancer or stops it cold from spreading in your body. At least not yet. But there are certain foods that qualify as prostate powerhouses at your table or on your menu:

Fiber: You get it from fruits, veggies, whole grains (look for 100 percent wheat on your bread labels, look for three or more grams per slice), beans and legumes. Here's what experts believe a high-fiber diet does: Binds to toxic carcinogens and other compounds later eliminated from the body; reduces hormone levels that can otherwise promote prostate cancer progression; and prompts blood serum changes in as little as 10 days when high-fiber consumption is combined with low intakes of saturated fat.

Here is what some studies suggest it might do: Reduce PSA values, and lower death rates among men who regularly include high-fiber cereals and nuts/seeds in their diets.

Cooked tomatoes: We are talking lycopene, a nutrient, (sheesh, it's even touted on ketchup bottles these days). Lycopene, which is released through heating tomatoes and their juices, is an antioxidant that scavenges unstable free radical cells, which in turn reduces tissue damage. There have been doubters about the effectiveness of lycopene, yet the research stacks up quite favorably for your tomato sauce, according to Lynn Goldstein, a dietitian who has counseled cancer patients at the Weill Medical College of Cornell University hospital in Manhattan and throughout the New York City area.

For example, in small studies, men who ate 30 milligrams of daily lycopene in the form of (regular servings of) tomato sauce for three weeks experienced a 28 percent reduction in oxidative DNA damage and an 18 percent drop in PSA levels. In terms of PSA, the men with prostate cancer who didn't eat the tomato sauce saw their levels rise 14 percent.

Some real-life info: Lycopene is better absorbed with some fat, such as a small amount of olive oil. The positive changes you can get with 30 daily milligrams can be measured as 4.5 tablespoons of tomato paste, 3/4 cup of tomato sauce, 12 ounces of tomato juice, or 8 medium raw tomatoes. Other sources of lycopene include watermelon (you need four cups for the daily 30 milligrams), grapefruit, papaya and guava.

PROSTATE POWERHOUSE FOODS: (PART II)

(GO SOY, GO FLAX, GO NUTS)

In health food circles, the drumbeat of soy-so-good-for-you can seem monotonous, at times. And that includes "magical" soybeans. But the fact remains that researchers believe soy as a staple is one shining reason why

Asian men have lower rates of prostate cancer than North Americans. The main chemical factor in soy appears to decrease male hormones in our blood serum that otherwise encourage prostate tumor growth. It also restricts enzymes in tumor growth and seems to act in ways that help to starve tumor cells. Figure to get one serving a day from soy foods—edamame (whole soybeans, in pods), tofu, tempeh, miso, soy nuts, soy milk—and skip the supplements.

Flaxseed: A number of studies have suggested flaxseed can block tumor growth while enhancing the immune system's ability to fight back. It also appears to bind with testosterone, which is a good thing for prostate cancer patients. There is evidence flax can help reduce the risk of metastasis and lead to less aggressive tumors.

Key note: Flax does contain alpha-linoleic acid or ALA, which has actually been associated with prostate cancer growth. But Natalie Ledesma and other cancer nutritionists point out that the "primary ALA sources in those studies were red meat, butter, mayonnaise and margarine."

You can get your daily flax serving with one to two tablespoons of flaxseed meal per day. Many patients buy flaxseed meal at standard grocery stories or buy seeds to grind themselves in a coffee bean grinder (we can't digest the hull of the seed, so eating them whole is not worthwhile). Also, the ground seeds need to be refrigerated. Try sprinkling the nutty-tasting flaxmeal over your cereal, or add it to a juice smoothie. Don't go to the expense of buying flax oil.

Brazil nuts: You know, the oversize nuts in cocktail mixes (that everyone leaves till last)—but they happen to be loaded with selenium. Studies show the mineral selenium inhibits cellular changes that can lead to prostate cancer; it can also lead to cancer cell death and decrease recurrences. A mere two Brazil nuts per day can provide a therapeutic 200 micrograms of selenium. (So long, Spanish peanuts!)

FISH LIST: "CATCH-AND-RELEASE" OMEGA-6

Any fish you wish? You have likely heard a lot of good-food news about omega-3 or "healthy" fats that are plentiful in cold-water fatty fish (salmon, sardines, freshwater trout, shellfish, anchovies), flaxseed, walnuts, canola oil and soybeans (try steaming frozen edamame (whole soybeans in the pods), salting them lightly, then popping the beans into your mouth and discarding the pods).

What you less about is the omega-6 overload in most all diets. Cancer nutritionist Natalie Ledesma says the typical U.S. man's diet has "way too much omega-6 fats" from processed foods and fried foods made with corn oil, safflower oil, cottonseed oil, soybean oil and other polyunsaturated oils. She recommends using olive oil for low-heat cooking and only canola or grapeseed oils for higher temperatures.

Most nutrition researchers estimate most men eat about two to five times more omega-6 fats than omega-3 fats. Ledesma wants her prostate patients shooting for a 1:1 ratio. She says there is considerable evidence that the linoleic acid in omega-6 fats can be converted to arachidonic acid that may stimulate the growth of prostate cancer cells, but admits other studies don't show the association.

Her take is decidedly not wait-and-see. Ledesma says to eat more omega-3 fats because it "limits the harm" of arachidonic acid. She especially urges men with aggressive prostate cancer to eat three or more fish meals per week. Naturally, she recommends broiling, grilling or even pan-frying in place of the deep fryer.

SHAKE, SHAKE, SHAKE

When Wall Street financier Michael Milken was diagnosed with advanced prostate cancer in 1993, he knew what he wasn't going to do. Doctors told him he had, oh, maybe a year to 18 months to live. One of his first thoughts was about Steven J. Ross, the former Time Warner chairman and a good friend who had died of prostate cancer just a month earlier.

"He [Ross] thought the idea of giving up eating the food you love is the same as giving you life," said Milken during a *New York Times* interview. But leading researchers even then were touting low-fat diets high in fruits, vegetables and soy for increased prostate cancer survival. Milken instantly changed his diet, along with undergoing aggressive treatments. He does admit that his eating during the treatment phase was "more of a burden than a pleasure."

This all changed, happily, when Milken met Beth Ginsberg, a personal chef who trained at the famed Culinary Institute of America in Napa Valley. "You can make healthy food taste like and look like the food you grew up with," she says. Between the two of them they devised recipes such as the Vegetable Reuben and (healthful) Devil's Fool Cake. Milken and Ginsberg authored *The Taste for Living Cookbook*, with all proceeds going to the Prostate Cancer Foundation, the powerful prostate cancer charity that Milken founded after his diagnosis.

One of Milken's most famed recipes, the Daily Soy Shake, appeared in *FORTUNE* magazine. Here's the sweet-tasting treat and pick-me-up—minus any of the simple table sugar that some cancer researchers associate with accelerated tumor growth. Try to add the cancer-fighter green tea when possible. The shake is a superb way to feed your sweet tooth and not your cancer cells.

MICHAEL MILKEN'S DAILY SOY SHAKE

* 1/2 cup organic pomegranate or mixed fruit juice
* 1/2 cup brewed organic green tea or other fruit juice
* 1/4 cup berries of your choice
* 1 banana
* 1 teaspoon grated lemon zest
* 1 teaspoon grated orange zest
* 1/2 cup strawberry-flavored or plain soy protein isolate powder

Directions: Place all ingredients in blender container and blend thoroughly.

Nutritional analysis per serving: 265 calories, 1.7 grams (g) fat, 0.2 g saturated fat, 0 g cholesterol, 22.1 g protein, 42 g carbohydrate, 3.3 g fiber, 207 milligrams sodium.

EXERCISING MORE CONTROL

There are dozens of good reasons for men to be physically active, even more as we grow older. For one, studies suggest that regular exercise habit —which can be as simple as walking and climbing stairs whenever the opportunity arises—play a positive role in preventing cancer. Reasons? The increased physical activity strengthens your immune system (including NK, or natural killer, cells), improves blood flow and accelerates the body's ability to digest food while eliminating toxins. And you've doubtless heard all the pluses of exercise against heart disease. Staying active is a way for men to feel in some control of their prostate diagnosis and recovery.

What's new about prostate cancer and exercise research is the expanding file of studies that show physical activity may lower the risk of an advanced diagnosis in men over 65. Here's a brief, but helpful, sampling: First, a 2005 study published in the *Annals of Internal Medicine*, for instance showed that men who pursued a vigorous exercise program were significantly less likely to receive Gleason scores at higher, riskier levels.

Second, lower mortality rates also were recorded for men who exercised at increasing levels of intensity, compared with a sedentary group, even when statisticians considered such key characteristics as body size, cigarettes smoked, family history of prostate cancer, diabetes, and diet, including tomato sauce consumption.

The Finish Line: An oft-quoted Harvard study from renowned epidemiologist Dr. Edward L. Giovannucci strongly suggests that, even among survivors, regular exercise can slow the progress of prostate cancer.

HOW THE GYM MAKES A STRONGER JIM

A related, ongoing study performed at the Ottawa (Canada) Health Research Institute shows that weight training can stave off fatigue while increasing muscle mass of men undergoing hormonal drug treatment. Fact is, androgen deprivation therapy will reduce a man's testosterone level, which does make the body a less-able host for tumor growth. But it typically knocks men for a hard-spinning loop. Survivors typically report feeling greater fatigue, less day-to-day function at work or home, weight gain and loss of muscle. Not a four-star scenario. Enter: The Ottawa scientists, who found that men who engaged in a moderate weight-lifting program for 12 weeks "had less interference" from fatigue during daily activities than the control group. Plus, the lifters improved both upper and lower body strength in before-and-after tests.

Here's an alluring thought from Anna Schwartz, a research associateprofessor at the University of Washington, who specializes in theeffects of physical activity during cancer treatment cycles. "You can actually get faster and stronger during treatment," she says. "Almost all patients feel better if they get up and move around a little bit. When you stay physically active you don't experience the physical decline [which gets worse the longer the radiation lasts]. Plus,exercise helps men on hormone therapy to counteract muscle loss and bone thinning."

Of course, feeling lousy or tired doesn't exactly make you want to jump into your walking or running togs. "Patients tell me all the time the most important time for them to exercise is when they feel their worst," says Schwartz.

ADULT SWIM (POST-OPERATIVE COMPETITION)

See if this sounds familiar to you or maybe a friend with prostate cancer: Healthy man, 69, goes into his annual physical feeling great. Doc says his PSA is up, enough to order a biopsy. Damn biopsy comes back positive. Doctor says watchful waiting is an option, as results don't appear to be aggressive.

The 69-year-old, no longer the picture of health in his mind's eye, seeks advice from doctors, friends, the Internet, the deli guy, about the best treatment choice. One pal in particular gets through to him. "Let me go introduce you to a friend who watched and waited," says the pal. "Great, OK, when?" asks the 69-year-old. "Any time," says the pal. "But we'll have to go to the cemetery."

That's when patient Bob Patten jumped in the pool. He ultimately decided on a laparoscopic radical prostatectomy or LRP, which is minimally invasive and which dramatically reduces recovery time. And we do mean "jumped in the pool." Patten is a Masters competitive swimmer. One day after the successful surgery (which produced "clear margins"), Patten went for a walk on a beach in the Miami area, where he had traveled to undergo the LRP with a leading practitioner. Patten refused any pain medications to ease the exercise. Some time during that walk, catheter tugging against him, Patten did some quick math and decision-making. He vowed to swim in the long-course nationals, just a hundred days away in August, 2004.

Patten jetted home to Denver with the catheter still attached. When docs tugged it out, 10 days after surgery, Patten dipped gently into his home pool at the Denver Athletic Club. He swam "easy" for 10 days, then started getting back into his usual rigorous laps and interval training for his preferred race, the breaststroke. Bob Patten trained six days a week in the pool and lifted weights (outside the pool). By the nationals event, he had turned 70, which bumped him into the next competing age group, 70 to 74 years old. Turns out he set an age group world record for the 200-meter breaststroke, crediting the LRP procedure as allowing him to fully recover and train.

Yet doctors won't take the credit, arguing that Patten's goal-setting and determination served him just as effectively. For the rest of us, there's a lot to be said for keeping active, even if it starts out as five minutes of walking in the morning and another five at night. Friends and competitors were not surprised by all the hoopla, even if Patten was caught off guard with his feat just a few splashes beyond three months of recovery.

"The meet announcer was saying a world record had been set," recalls Patten, laughing, during an interview with *Swimming World Magazine*, "and I'm looking around to see who beat me."

100 WISE WORDS FROM A WORLD-CLASS FOOD & FITNESS GURU

When we heard Walter Willett, M.D., Ph.D., professor of medicine at Harvard Medical School and the Harvard School of Public Health, and author of the amazingly sensible, *Eat, Drink and Be Healthy*, was going to give a talk about nutrition and cancer at the 2006 ASCO (American Society of Clinical Oncology) annual meeting, we put down our tortilla chips and applied for a press pass at the convention—even if it was scheduled for Atlanta in the pre-summer steamy heat. Once arrived, we grabbed a front row seat. The man, no matter what you may think of his (food) politics or nearly erect, near-fu-manchu moustache, knows his food and fitness, and speaks with more than 35 years of top-shelf dietary research and practice embedded in his brain. Plus, at 60, he still bikes his butt to work two miles every day (as he has for decades) instead of driving.

In his mid-morning ASCO talk, which ranged from general cautions ("There's really no doubt that... obesity is related to cancer risk," and "Maybe the effects of diet [on risks] are more important in early life.") to specifics like telling men they should ingest more Vitamin D—plus drink less milk—to reduce prostate and other cancer risks, Willett mowed through decades of research in less than an hour. In this, a chapter on diet, we thought it would be helpful to do even more reducing: So here are 100 of Walter Willett's wisest words on the matter of healthful eating and exercise.

"The potential impact of healthy diet, when you combine it with not smoking and regular physical activity, is enormous. For example, our studies have shown that we could prevent about 82 percent of heart attacks, about 70 percent of strokes, over 90 percent of type 2 diabetes, and over 70 percent of colon cancer, with the right dietary choices as part of a healthy lifestyle. The best drugs can reduce heart attacks by about 20 or 30 percent, yet we put almost all of our resources into promoting drugs rather than healthy lifestyle and nutrition." *

Oops. Seems that's only 95 words. So, professor Willett, is it true you believe exercise, not calorie– or carb-counting, should be at the core of everyone's lifestyle?

"Right." says he. "Exercise is absolutely essential."

*PBS *Frontline* report, 4/8/04

WALK-TALK FOR LONG LIFE

It seems like a simple act, putting one foot in front of the other.For most of us, for most of our lives, it is.

But survivors repeatedly look back at their first walks down a hospital hallway, or maybe their backyard or a beach (like Bob Patten, above) as marker moments, once they'd heard a diagnosis or underwent surgery. The vital strategy is to keep those feet moving during any treatment choice. For Simon & Schuster publishing exec and author Michael Korda, his daily post-op walk was the consistent and trusted talisman in his recovery from a frightening bout with prostate cancer. Consider this passage from his achingly honest, 1996 memoir, *Man to Man*:

"I believed absolutely...that my walk, lengthened every day, taken every day even when the temperature plummeted (one morning was so cold that the urine in my bag froze solid; it made no difference, we went on) was what ultimately saved me from despair, fueled my recovery and brought me back...."

No matter the season, no matter the climate, call it exercise as medicine once more.

THE 19TH HOLE

One of the best ways to fit in a walk is to play golf—without a cart. While the possibility of impotence or incontinence weighs on a man's mind while choosing treatments (and most every day through recovery), there remains the still-relevant question for many patients: "Hey, what's gonna happen to my golf game?"

Dr. Mitchell Benson, chairman of urology at Columbia University College of Physicians and Surgeons and a decent golfer himself, decided one day to semi-formally address the question. He decided to follow 55 men with prostate cancer who underwent radical prostatectomies, by asking them about their golf handicap before the surgery, whether their golf performance improved or worsened after surgery—and why, if applicable, they thought there was a change. As it turned out, 36 of the men—or 60 percent—reported their games actually improved post-operatively. These three dozen men dropped their handicaps by an average of three strokes, attributing the improvement to a slower and more rhythmic swing, mostly from fear that swinging too hard would lead to incontinence, or leaks at the tee. Only eight of the men said their swings and games got worse for the same reason—believing they scored higher, for fears of an onset of incontinence while out on the course. Least they didn't blame their putter.

CHAPTER 5

Bedroom, Bathroom, Intimacy Notes

Curtis Pesmen

"Would you like to be less of a man?"

Would anybody? With all the talk-talk-talk about treatments and side effects and life-after-prostate cancer, that's the question that goes unspoken before a doctor goes to work on your testosterone-fueled tumor(s). For starters as to why, there's no easy way to ask such a thing. So he may ask "around" it. As in: "What's most important to you about the operation or treatment...?" (Or as Vietnam-era vets remember too well, "Sometimes we have to burn the village to save the village.") Second, part of any good doc's job is to reassure you, to help you heal in both psychological and physical ways, following a major trauma.

So even when all goes well with surgery, seeds, radiation and the

> **"When my catheter came out, I was totally incontinent. I had to wear a diaper for five months. I'm a lawyer; I'd be in court...and could feel myself leaking."**
>
> —Survivor, 61, as told to *Best Life* magazine

resultant PSA, there may well be hurdles in healing that chip away a man's dignity. Time and again. Might start with the predicted post-op physio-sorts of stuff, from simple to complex pain. Might then move along to day-to-day survivor subjects like anxiety, fatigue, blood in the urine (or semen) or urinary incontinence; then finally move forward to other issues of the bedroom, as in erections or non-erections, and into matters of the mind—and manhood.

BEDROOM NOTES:

AN UNFAIR CHOICE?

"I chose surgery, although I [was told] the likelihood of impotence or incontinence is about 30 to 40 percent," relates a relatively young survivor, James R., of Milwaukee, now nearing age 60. "My doctor asked me prior to surgery if I wanted him, during surgery, to mainly be concerned about doing the utmost to eliminate all possibility of cancer...or did he want me to have him try to give me the best chance to avoid impotence, by not cutting the nerves [astride the gland]. I said, 'Living cancer-free is my top priority.' I would accept the impotence, if necessary.

"There's always the chance it would come back, and new drugs are coming out all the time.... I was cut—and as a result I haven't been able to get an erection," says James. "I will never know if another surgeon could have avoided cutting the [main] nerve, or if it would have made any difference." Unemotional bottom line: James R. is cancer-free. James is erection-free.

OTHER HURDLES IN HEALING

The psychological hurts inflicted by prostate cancer are almost too numerous to name. Yet those related to intimacy often cut deeper. "I don't want to talk about it," is a common first thought; first course of action for many survivors. Which is understandable. But it's also one reason why I, a colon cancer survivor—and countless prostate cancer survivors—are unhappy to read such pro-forma, gloomy forecasts as the following, which often are posted in a prominent places for prostate patients and their families to read:

"Loss of desire may result from worry and depression, nausea or pain," one Internet report reported (too matter-of-factly for my taste). Of course loss of desire will result from this threat to a man's life—and manhood. This felt patronizing to me, however true it may be.   "After treatment...there may still be little interest in sex." Again, totally under-standable. Then comes the understatement of understatements: "Cancer treatments that disturb the normal hormone balance can also lessen sexu-al desire." No kidding. (see chart below, "Sexual Side Effects...") Many or most prostate hormone treatments are designed to shut down the testi-cles, at least temporarily. That'll have a "lessening" effect, for sure. It's not the message that's the problem here: It's the lack of framework pro-vided to patients who, indeed, "may not want to talk about it." We'll try to provide some necessary framework throughout this chapter.

PROSTATE MAP (PART I)

A URETHRA RUNS THROUGH IT

You could call it fraction—or in-fraction—time: For the first half of a man's life, the prostate gland is mostly about sex, reproduction and, well, sex. Its growth stimulated by testosterone hormone from the testicles, the prostate manufactures milky prostatic fluid that joins the sperm and sends semen, the life-affirming stuff of men upward, onward, outward. For the second half of life, the prostate is more about aging, annoyance and at times well-grounded fear. Nestled low in the pelvis, beneath the pubic cradle of bone, the prostate is shish-kabobbed between the penis and bladder. In place of a skewer, though, the urethra runs through it, carry-ing urine, most of the time, but also semen when the time is right. And forget, the latest experts say, all the talk about the prostate being a walnut, or walnut-sized, whatever. (Guess we could lose the shish-kabob reference, too.) It's more helpful and realistic, docs suggest, to consider the prostate as a plumb, especially as it is pliable, red, and prone to all sorts of shape-shifting over time.

As a quick reminder, urologists won't hesitate a second to explain to many middle-aged and older men that, well, a rising PSA could mean many things besides cancer, including relatively harmless BPH—benign prostatic hyperplasia—which is not much more than age-related swelling of the gland to the point where it pinches the urethra and causes a number of nagging, urination-related complaints. But cancer it ain't.

These days, no matter the treatment method, urologists and oncologists say their goals have been refined. Better mapping of the gland, and of your condition, leads to better long-term results and "HRQOL" (as they also say), or Health-Related Quality of Life. In post-2005 treatment plans, medical teams typically talk about setting more precise targets for radiation beams, seeds or scalpels, with less damage from friendly fire. At a recent prostate cancer conference run by the American Society of Clinical Oncology (ASCO), I sat in on a packed-hotel-ballroom talk by Anthony Zeitman, M.D., an Oxford- and Harvard-trained doc, who at one point told his audience, "We need better prostate imaging, and more accurate radiation delivery systems. You need to see your target, and have better aim—" at which point an oversized photo of Vice President Dick Cheney coolly popped onscreen inside Dr. Zeitman's PowerPoint presentation, eliciting unplanned laughs from the thousand-plus doctors in attendance. Seems they'd recently heard of Veep Cheney's unfortunate, human-to-human hunting accident down on the ranch.

PROSTATE MAP (PART II)

NERVES RUN THROUGH IT

For a surgeon or radiation oncologist, for all the reasons above, the cancerous prostate is never an easy target. To make matters more complicated, the "arms" of the gland carry microscopic—but critical to sexual pleasure—nerves and blood vessels that help make erections erect. When these are burned by radiation or sliced by a scalpel, amid an often bloody "field" during surgery, a man's capacity for sexual performance takes a huge hit, sometimes irreversible. "I was cut...," we recall James R. saying, meaning a very tiny, but important, part of his erectile anatomy was severed during prostatectomy.

On the other hand, newish nerve-sparing surgery (see Chapter 3) doesn't always mean you're going to be potent for life, either. A key factor in the prognoses that patients don't always hear has to do with the quality of erections—both before and after surgery. In short, by the time a man reaches 55, his normal, healthy (unaided by drug) erections don't have the force, turgidity and feel of those he had when he was 25. Truth is, they are softer and less-rapidly aroused. No world-class expertise in prostate surgery alone can undo the vascular and nerve changes that normally accompany aging (or certain age-related diseases).

Instead, the prospect of high-quality, nerve-sparing surgery or pinpoint seed placement merely ups your odds of facing lesser negative effects. Yet these improved odds are worth considering--a prime reason why second or third opinions matter. After being treated for prostate cancer, for the most part no matter the method, your sexual equip-ment will remind you, often at first and hopefully much less later, that it has undergone medical trauma. For survivors, one oft-overlooked goal is to reduce that trauma throughout the first, or second, course of treatment. It's not enough any longer to say, gruffly, "I want my prostate on someone's shelf."

There's such a thing, hard-to-believe, as being too aggressive for your own good while treating cancer. It's a balancing act, with your input required. As Dr. Zeitmen appeared to suggest to his urologic-oncologist colleagues at the San Francisco Marriott in early 2006: "Sometimes you don't have to burn the village to save the village." Truth is, the fields of prostate and nerve mapping, plus medical imaging, are advancing rapidly and in dozens of new, hopeful directions. But they still may remain, in regard to your particu-lar prostate treatment, imprecise

SEXUAL SIDE EFFECTS OF TREATMENTS

Powerful treatment often coincides with prolonged or unexpected effects. In prostate cancer, here are the some of the most widely cited sexual side effects, as summarized by and adapted from the American Cancer Society (www.cancer.org).

TREATMENT	LOW SEX DESIRE	ERECTION PROBLEMS	LACK OF ORGASM	DRY ORGASM	WEAKER ORGASM	INFERTILITY
RADICAL PROSTATEC-TOMY	Rarely	Often	Rarely	Always	Sometimes	Always
RADIATION THERAPY (PELVIC)	Rarely	Sometimes	Rarely	Rarely	Sometimes	Often
HORMONE THERAPY	Often	Often	Sometimes	Sometimes	Sometimes	Always
ORCHIECTOMY (TESTES REMOVED)	Often	Often	Sometimes	Sometimes	Sometimes	Always
CHEMO-THERAPY*	Sometimes	Rarely	Rarely	Rarely	Sometimes	Often

*Note: Certain chemotherapy drugs may prevent emission, causing retrograde ejaculation of sperm (into bladder).

SEPTUAGENARIAN SEXUAL SIDE EFFECTS

When my dad, at 75, decided to opt for radiation and hormones to vanquish his early-stage prostate cancer, he knew it was a long-haul treatment. Still, he later fell into a kind of funk. For a time he pulled back from those closest to him, including my mother and sister, and we wondered what was "wrong." Trauma, not impotence concerns, was what was wrong. Plus fear. Plus joint and severe back pain—back pain he blamed in part on the hormones that he believes sapped his bones of strength. Plus fatigue. Plus the realization that he would be a patient, of sorts, for the rest of his life.

And I think, truth be told, he felt cheated: Till this cancer arrived, he still felt "young" for his age. For both his parents lived into their mid-90s, and here he was, post-radiation, in his 70s, walking the aisles of a drugstore, shopping for incontinence pads that his doctors warned he might need to use, for weeks, or possibly months, to come. (Come to think of it, this, too can tend to do a number on a man's sexual confidence.)

One note I'd found in the medical literature and thought of sending to my dad, as a kind of gentle warning, said, "Any thought that keeps a man from feeling excited can also interfere with his getting or keeping an erection." Then I decided against sending it, because I felt I'd be invading his privacy. He had, in fact, a license to be angry. (Thinking back, I recalled my normally jocular father didn't seem too thrilled to receive, from a friend, a complimentary dose of Viagra for his 75th birthday, along with a suitably sarcastic birthday card. Yet I was—and remain—curious about the source of the drug, as his friend was—and is—over the age of 80.)

Sexually speaking, even without worrying about prostate cancer and treatment, a man in midlife or older has had a few things on his mind in recent years. Among most every man of a certain age—sexually active or semi-active—one of the first signs of age-related change—beyond erection quality—is in his "ejaculatory inevitability" (a fine phrase, otherwise known as "coming"), which is less sharp, more diffuse, and tends to be slightly less pleasurable. Again, this is not caused by prostate cancer, or even BPH, but is better to know about in one's 40s and 50s than to learn about it later, maybe surprisingly, in a frustrating session in bed.

WHEN PENISES SHRINK: WHAT PATIENTS AND DOCS THINK (PART I)

It was a show-stopping quote; one I'll not soon forget. And it had more to do with the penis than the prostate: Celestia Higano, M.D., of the University of Washington, was at the podium, speaking to hundreds of doctors at the ASCO Prostate Cancer Symposium, in February, 2006, about better hormone ("anti-androgen") treatments, and ways to improve prostate cancer patient care, when she read from a patient's journal without apology, medicalese, or any kind of censorship.

"We don't see what patients often report," she told her fellow docs, and began to excerpt the account, "written by a patient, from a journal... I don't normally read: 'My mental and physical vigor have deserted me,' [the patient wrote]. 'I started developing breasts and gaining weight, particularly in my backside, like a woman.

'My penis has shrunk. It's dead. In fact it's been lost between my thighs, which have grown enormous. I find it hard [to look at my wife].'

Dr. Higano wasn't trying to chastise her audience. She merely was trying to call for better survivorship care, including more complete pre and post-op, and pre- and post-treatment information sessions about what changes are expected to occur in the body throughout a full course of treatment.

SEX AND MY CANCER, REVISITED

A few years ago, when I was a Stage III colorectal cancer patient prepping for major surgery, down deep in my pelvic cavity, where the rectum nearly nudges the prostate, I had a talk with one of my surgeons. Turned out my main colon and rectal surgeon, Mark Lane Welton, M.D., wanted to "bring in the cavalry" to help him out, including Peter Carroll, M.D., the chairman of the department of urology at the University of California-San Francisco's medical and cancer centers. "He's going to help me stay out of the prostate," Dr. Welton says. Sounded okay to me, especially as I knew that Dr. Carroll recently had operated—and successfully—upon the cancerous prostate of Robert Mueller, now director of our F.B.I.

Stay out of the prostate, indeed. The way I saw it, it's not enough lousy luck that I—Mr. Health Book Author—get colorectal cancer at age 43, that I'm going to have my abdominal organs rearranged. Now one of the top urologic surgeons in the country is telling me, after reviewing the MRI scan of my pelvis, that in surgery I may lose some of the nerves that help erections become erections. Without those nerves, bundled around the prostate and hideously close to the rectum, I understand in a hurry, I may soon be Viagra-dependent, sexually speaking.

"We just want the cancer out," my noble wife Paula tells Dr. Carroll. I think, "Maybe we want a little more than that."

WHEN PENISES SHRINK: WHAT PATIENTS AND DOCS THINK (PART II)

For the record, Dr. Higano (above) also reported: "In regard to a decrease in penile and testicular size, althought it's variable and not well studied, up to 68 percent of men have penile shortening after radical prostatecomy [surgery]."

In fact, this was the second time I'd heard about the surprise of shrunken penises within the space of a six weeks. Jim Kiefert, an Us,TOO support group leader and two-time survivor first diagnosed in 1989, alerted me to the fact that penises shrink during prostate cancer surgery, after a portion of ure-thra has been snipped out, along with the diseased prostate. The ends of the urethra that remain are pulled and stitched together during the operation, but like a busted shoelace, it's never the same length once you've knotted together the loose ends. We know this about shoelaces. But not about post-op penises. Even in the late 2000s, I am told, too many men aren't warned about this key side effect, before undergoing prostate cancer surgery.

5 KEY QUESTIONS ABOUT SEX EFFECTS

Q1. "CAN I STILL HAVE SEX AFTER SURGERY? IF SO, HOW SOON?"

Yes, with a few caveats. While it makes sense to revert to your former lifestyle where possible, it also makes sense to not hurry. And make certain your internist or cardiologist is aware of your "return." So take your time, experts advise. At four weeks post-op, in the best of cases, urologists will tell otherwise healthy post-op prostate cancer patients, "Okay, go for it."

Q2. "EVER HAVE A DRY ORGASM?"

Mike Carlson, a Wisconsin patient who chose radioactive seed therapy in 1998 at the Mayo Clinic in Rochester, Minnesota, was talking with a friend who also faced prostate cancer in recent years: "I talked with one of my ski-ing buddies who had surgery," Carlson says, "and asked him what his sex life was like after the operation. He said, 'Ever have the dry heaves?'" Translation: orgasm without ejaculation. (Or, rather, retrograde ejaculation, which sends sperm back into the bladder instead of out the penis.) It's something that takes some getting used to, post-op patients explain. But for many men, the sensations—and pleasurable waves—of orgasm remain.

Q3. "WHEN IS SEX 'NOT QUITE' SEX?"

Oftentimes, during survivorship. Another instance, according to Terry Real, a family therapist in Cambridge, Massachusetts, and author of *I Don't Want to Talk About It*, is when people are feeling undue pressures about major life events. These pressures, which can arise during financial upheaval and other major disruptions, can lead to unexpected and uncomfortable moments in bed. Even between eager, compatible sex partners.

"His nerves may cause him to seek sex when all he really wants is reassurance or some support from his partner." Real explained in an interview. "It's just that he may find it easier to reach out for that support under the covers late at night rather than in the kitchen, face-to-face. He may want to talk, but what he knows to do is grab her in bed."

Q4: WHY DOES SEX (AND PEEING) FEEL LESS PLEASURABLE THAN BEFORE?

It doesn't always. However, if certain tissues around the prostate are scarred by surgery or radiation, there may be a two- or three-stage side effect of damage to your sex and excretionary equipment. Some changes are felt immediately after treatment; these are predictable. Less predictable are the short- and long-term effects of damaged cells and tissues that doctors can't even see. Radiation damage, for instance, may not fully set in for weeks, months or years.

Then, too, some researchers, including one I interviewed at Northwestern University Medical School in Chicago, have linked pleasurable feelings during urination to a "U-Spot" (U for urethra), of sorts, that is rich with nerves and capable of stirring reportedly strong sexual feeling. This observation (related to treatment effects) hasn't been widely reported in the media—or even in the most complete patient brochures. Call it also "U," for under-reported.

Q5: WHAT IF I CAN'T TAKE VIAGRA, LEVITRA or CIALIS?

The new erectile-dysfunction drugs may be powerful, but they also may not be for everyone. If your doctor doesn't think it wise for you to use them, you might remind yourself—as sex therapists often do—that a man's most powerful sex organ isn't the penis, testicles or prostate: It's the brain. The second most powerful, then? The skin. Neither of which are harmed irrevocably by even the most powerful prostate cancer drugs.

BATHROOM, INTIMACY NOTES:

URINE TROUBLE

It's hard to say which of these three numbers is most important: 1) 3 pads a day. Some doctors, for research reasons, don't consider post-op patients to be "incontinent" if they use three or fewer incontinence pads a day. 2) 1 urine-soaked spot on the floor of a $50,000 auto import. 3) 14 percent of men still suffered urine leakage five years after prostate cancer surgery, according to a May, 2005, *Journal of Urology* study of nearly 1,300 men.

From a survivor's or patient's point of view, it's the second number, the urine-soaked spot in the car that drives the point home. Incontinence due to prostate cancer causes layers of problems; not just the temporary (for most) trouble that follows patients home from the hospital.

Writing about the early stages of this problem in his book, *Man to Man*, survivor Michael Korda recalls a New York City night in which his prostate forced him to pull off the busy West Side Highway, "Traffic streamed by.... I felt a confused mixture of shame, guilt and fear at my loss of control, coupled with inexpressible physical relief as I emptied my bladder in full sight of the world."

Fortunately, post-operatively, a couple hundred pages later Korda (whom I was fortunate enough to interview) was able to stash away the Depends and write, "Sir Dignity Briefs looked like normal underwear, and felt normal, too."

BEAST OF BURDEN

Like Korda, tens of thousands of prostatectomy survivors have found in recent years that temporary leakage is one thing; but that persistent, long-term urine leakage is another matter entirely. Patients say, time and again, that incontinence trumps impotence in terms of its many burdens...and what it takes to manage the condition daily. According to reliable, national patient surveys published by the Us TOO support group, from 39 to 63 percent of patients report they are still incontinent one year after surgery. What's more, reports say 24 to 56 percent of those patients were wearing incontinence pads one year after their surgery.

DO THE MATH: 25 X 2 = BETTER URINATION

For men, it's new math. Yet women have known of them—Kegel exercises—for years (and not just for post-childbirth genital health). Performed quickly, stealthily, 25 times, twice each day, Kegels can strengthen a few key muscles that interact with messenger nerves along the urinary pathways. Kegels, or pelvic muscle exercises, also are prescribed to singles and couples in sex therapy, in search of stronger orgasms. The sought-after, six-week result: Stronger, more youthful musculature inside the pelvis, that supports the bladder and prostate and leads to better, stronger, more obedient urinary control. And, we hope, better orgasms for both partners.

Here's how to perform, and squeeze them in: Start by squeezing, pausing, then releasing, the muscles that you use to "hold" urination, about 15 times, twice each day. You can do them at home, in a car, in an office: No one else will know. After a couple weeks, do 25 Kegels twice a day, and begin to hold the "hold" for a second or two longer. (Some people swear by 50 or 75 a day, but we're being realistic here.)

Bonus: While Kegels or pelvic muscle workouts are a discussion staple at prostate support group meetings for improving incontinence (or in the brochures handed out at them), Dr. Bernie Zilbergeld, author of The New Male Sexuality, tells readers the payoff, whatever the math involved, is in "increasing orgasm intensity."

Rx'S TO REGAIN URINARY CONTROL

All incontinence drugs are not created equal(ly). In fact, some, like anti-depressants, weren't created for incontinence at all—yet they work for many survivors, just the same. This is a tricky task, however; using perfectly legal drugs for "off-label" uses, because in this instance, doctors know there may be other medical issues at hand beside the incontinence. Yet when the medications work, and safely, doctors will find ways to let patients in on the good news.

In the rundown below, some Rx's act on the bladder to relax its muscles; others tighten those muscles or urethra muscles. Here's a brief look at some of the most commonly prescribed medications for regaining control, following prostate cancer treatment. For safety, remember to bring all your medical records to the table, as certain pre-existing conditions, like hypertension or diabetes, will pre-empt certain choices from your doc's list of tried-and-true possibilities.

STRESS Incontinence	URGE Incontinence	OVERFLOW Incontinence
Decongestants include prescribed and over-the-counter brands to tighten urethral muscles (e.g., during a cough).	For urge incontinence, anticholinergic agents – oxybutynin (Ditropan), hyoscyamine (Levbid, Cytospaz), or tolterodine (Detrol) are often prescribed to relax overactive bladder muscles. This in turn delays the urge to urinate and allows the bladder to hold more urine.	For overflow incontinence (a dripping of urine), many doctors are prescribing antiadrenergics such as prazosin (Minipress), terazosin (Hytrin) or doxazosin (Cardura).
Tricyclic antidepressants (used short term to tighten bladder neck muscles) include: imipramine (Tofranil) and amitriptyline (Vanatrip, Elavil, Endep).		

POST-OP INDIGNITY (PART I)

Nope, didn't have prostate cancer. (Least not yet; though it runs in the family.) Had colon cancer surgery instead, down in my rectum; hard by the prostate, almost touching it, matter of fact. Barely millimeters away, according to the high-resolution CT scan of my cancerous tumor.... Which is one reason why things weren't so clean, during and after...the Big Cut: my eight-hour surgery, in which a prostate cancer surgeon co-piloted my colorectal surgeon. What took so long? Cancer isn't easy, to be brief. Quite a production, as I recall (and as I scrawled in my journal); with more than a few side effects, or "EFX," in the parlance of Hollywood.

INTERIOR: Darkened Bedroom, 5:30 a.m., camera push [WIFE's P.O.V.] into HUSBAND [me] rolling slowly out of bed.

CUT TO: Int. bathroom dimly lit, mirror shot reveals HUSBAND standing in front of toilet with doughnut-sized ring of pee on Calvin Klein boxers.

"Son...of...a...bitch," is all I could think, after all the chemo and radiation and eight-hour-complicated surgery. "Body, don't break down on me now...." Waking up pre-dawn to pee, easing my post-surgical aching body, face up, off the bed into upright position with strategic use of elbow power and knee leverage (I look and feel like a damn Dungeness crab), and flicking on the bathroom light: Something's wrong. There, on my gray cotton underwear, to the right of where my penis resides, is a spot, a wet spot, bigger than a quarter, a lot bigger than a quarter. My eyes lock in on the spot, or rather the reflection of the spot in the bathroom mirror. I don't believe it: After what I've been through, from life-threatening diagnosis at 43, through chemo-radiation, bone-racking pain to setbacks and major, life-saving surgery, now I've got to suffer the indignity of a leaking dick? This is not what I ordered....

POST-OP INDIGNITY (PART II)

Not quite 12 hours after my near-bedwetting episode , my surgeons have slipped me into their schedules to see what's up, bladderwise. Did they nick a urogenital nerve by mistake, somewhere during my surgery? No time to ponder possibilities I have no clue about; it's time to piss into a "Flowmeter" contraption in the urology clinic, a spinning disc beneath a large funnel, set up atop a toilet that measures urine volume and force of the ...s-t-r-e-a-m. These are things I've never had checked before, as I'm not a 78-year-old, with a history of urination troubles. But I whip it out, hit the target, and watch a needle record my "output."

Then it's flush, wash up, and hop over to the ultrasound room, where Nurse Dora squirts cold jelly on my belly—"Watch the incision stitches," I plead—and she starts pressing on me with a wand as she looks for the grainy shadows of my bladder onscreen. Seems at first glance I'm "emptying okay;" seems that my stop/start mechanisms of urination are in working order as well. For now, docs think the trouble's not uromechanical, not in my penis or bladder or muscles therein, but actually a side effect: As I'm still healing from my surgery, still popping 17 pain pills round the clock, I'm sleeping better, longer, more soundly than I've slept in months. And as the pain eases each week, the narcotics I've been prescribed apparently put me under so deeply that I don't feel the first inner twinges of taking a piss that normally would wake a man like me in the wee hours of the morning. After all, docs point out, the urine leaking isn't happening during the day when I'm awake (as it does with many prostate cancer patients.)...

Feeling better now, about half of my excretionary equipment, feeling that even though my colon and rectum were downsized, maybe I won't need bladder surgery to fix my powers of urination. Unfortunately, I'm supposed to make a follow-up appointment with the Masters of Urologic Plumbing. Unfortunately, I'll be...back.

BIOFEEDBACK VS. PENILE CLAMPS

Whether you call them penile, or penis clamps, or External Urethral Compression Devices (EUCDs), it's hard to argue with their rates of success. For a certain amount of time at least, penile clamps do what they promise. Using straps, or rigid, flexible structures, they slip over the penis and, through pressure, help you hold it, and stay dry longer. When prescribed by a doctor, many are reimbursed by health insurance firms or Medicare.

Clamps are inexpensive, relatively simple to use, readily available. There are two major types: rigid/semi-rigid and strap types. Rigid clamps have a plastic or metal frame whose shape cannot be altered; semi-rigid clamps have a malleable (bendable) metal frame. Strap type clamps, as is evident by their name, consist of a flexible strap. Most clamps have a specially designed ridge, or hump, the presses on the urethra, thus preventing urine from flowing to the outside of the body.

At the same time, biofeedback and (nurse-taught) bladder control techniques may offer more appeal to survivors afflicted with more minor or temporary urinary problems. These behavioral techniques, incorporating mind/body matters of control, take time to learn, and success rates vary over a standard, 10-session course. But biofeedback—using monitors and displays and electrodes affixed to body parts—offers patients incremental rewards and a solid chance to regain control over at least part of their lost urinary control.

FOLLOW THE MONEY, THE INCOME STREAM, THE URINE STREAM

Sometimes money talks louder than any doctor or website. Not long ago, I came across a report on incontinence in the *American Journal of Nursing*—a magazine I don't read very often—that stopped me cold. I had to read one sentence in it twice:

"An estimated 3.4 million men over the age of 60 are affected—in fact, Medicare costs for treatment of urinary incontinence in men older than 65 have doubled since 1992."

Doubled, since 1992. And the last time I checked, the total annual cost of urinary incontinence for men in the United States (in 1995 dollars) was estimated at $3.8 billion (vs. $12.4 billion for women), according to a study in *Obstetrics and Gynecology* (2001), another magazine that writes about the body monthly but isn't quite as sexy a read as my monthly *GQ*.

This tells me that the frustration I have heard in some docs' voices at medical conferences; the frustration I've heard while listening to prostate cancer patients speak at support groups; and the frustration I've heard from the wives of recovering prostate cancer patients is all tip-of-the-iceberg stuff. Gentlemen, we have a problem. It's a silent epidemic of sorts—one that's at once embarrassing, painful, irritating, costly and severely underreported.

Remember the survivor's words at the top of this chapter? I, especially as an ex-cancer patient who had to submit to a kind of colostomy in search of a cure, won't soon forget them: "When my catheter came out," he said. "I was totally incontinent. I had to wear a diaper for five months. I'm a lawyer; I'd be in court...and could feel myself leaking."

Throughout these pages, we've brought light to patients in various throes of suffering or recovery. We've probably not focused enough on the day-to-day struggles that prostate cancer survivors and patients face in silence and, wrongly, in shame. The hope for the future—near-term and long-term is that, like AIDS and breast cancer advocates have done since the 1980s, prostate cancer advocates and patients, along with their medical staffs and industry leaders, will begin to treat urinary incontinence as a pandemic; not as an afterthought.

RESOURCES

For further personal, reliable information on incontinence, impotence and related issues, consider reaching:

1) **Us TOO International Inc.**, services and support groups. Downers Grove, IL (630) 795-1002   <www.ustoo.org>

2) **Prostate Cancer Foundation** Santa Monica, CA (800) 757-CURE (2873) <www.prostatecancerfoundation.org> (click on "side effects," "urinary dysfunction," "erectile dysfunction" at bottom of screen)

3) **People Living With Cancer**, an ASCO website, run and overseen by the American Society of Clinical Oncology. Contact ASCO (703) 797-1914 <www.plwc.org>

4) **The Prostate Net**, patient support and program services. (888) 477-6763 <www.prostate-online.com>

INTIMACY OF A DIFFERENT SORT
"Would you like to live with more of a man?"

Maureen Kiefert never had that question put to her exactly. But as the wife of the (two-time survivor and) chairman of the Us TOO International prostate cancer support group, she has seen her husband, Jim, face prostate surgery, recovery, then a second round of advanced hormone treatment over the course of 17 years. She still marvels at his grace—and power—through his steady battles, including a recent round of monthly infusions of Zometa, which controls bone cancer. It's not daily, predictable sexual activity this couple is after, it's closeness, love and intimacy of a different sort.

"Mentally and spiritually, [Jim] couldn't be better," Maureen said not long ago. "His energy certainly has not declined. How can you be with someone who is positive all the time and not pick up on it...? He exhibits his true self as he hugs our family and friends and as he holds my hand on our daily walks. As for me, I am along for this ride of a lifetime. He has taught me so much, and we continue to learn from each other."

"It's such an attack on masculinity," Jim told me shortly after the ASCO prostate cancer meeting in 2006. "The other cancers have devastating effects, but for a male to go through erectile dysfunction, and the possibility of incontinence, by God. It just takes away your dignity."

This is powerful stuff; perhaps as powerful as the female-like hormone treatments that have pumped through Maureen's husband Jim...that somehow, along with extending his life markedly, have made him more of a man.

CHAPTER 6

Holistic Health Help: Herbs and Natural Agents

Bob Condor

For days, Danny Dover and his wife, Mary, could barely talk to each other. Danny had just received about the worst 50th birthday present a guy could get. His urologist called with positive results on his prostate biopsy.

"The news just exploded in my head," recalls Danny, who is the piano technician at Dartmouth College (NH). "My father died five years earlier of the same disease. It felt as if the world I knew was caving in and I was going to die, it was that simple."

And frightening. The urologist quickly recommended surgery or radiation. Danny did his research and turned up more uncertainty about which was the best choice than he cared to accept. He was surprised there was no "compelling evidence" to choose one of the treatments over "simply

"On his own, [Michael] Milken decided to change his diet radically to one devoid of fat.... He added meditation, sesame oil massages, armoatherapy and yoga."

—from a *FORTUNE* cover story, Nov. 29, 2004

doing nothing." Danny's instincts led him to Internet support sites and for-midable encouragement from survivors about holistic therapies, including one man who called Danny from Japan. Danny was heartened but still spin-ning. Mary stepped in with an important name: Dr. Susan Kowalsky, a naturopathic physician practicing in their area. Danny liked her, saw Dr. Kowalsky as "the bridge I was looking for."

The naturopathic doc suggested supplements and dietary changes, detox fasting, bodywork, stress reduction, exercise and even dental work to help repair the immune system (anecdotally, some survivors report lower PSA levels after dental problems such as gum disease or decaying teeth are addressed).

Sitting right there in Dr. Kowalsky's office during the first visit, Danny and Mary started crying from relief and "all the tension we had been carrying." "Suddenly I was in the driver's seat," says Danny. "I would be responsible for my own healing and [Dr. Kowalsky] was there to help as needed."

Danny felt back in control of his life.

Six years later, he feels healthier than at any time in the last two decades. He continues to monitor his PSA levels for any indication of cancer growth.

That's what holistic or natural therapies can do for prostate cancer patients. They can give men and their families not just hope—but a sense of accom-plishment, while trying positive steps (and while watching and waiting), get-ting ready for surgery or recovering from radiation cycles. Holistic or inte-grative medicine treatments can help you regain a sense of control, howev-er piecemeal, after a shock diagnosis knocks you speechless and numb.

Throughout this chapter, you'll find a thoughtful sampling of the most advanced holistic medicine treatments—and techniques—that may indeed keep you strong—and in control.

THAT'S THE TRUTH, DOC

A recent study shows that about quarter of prostate cancer patients in the U.S. turn to complementary or integrative therapies, mostly dietary supplements. The percentage is about the same in the United Kingdom, where herbal remedies have long been accepted as part of medical treatment. Interestingly, about half the men on both shores (43 percent) did not inform their doctors of their supplement regimens. This is a mistake. While those patients likely are looking to avoid the verbal static they might hear from some doctors ("it's not proven," "you are wasting your money," "might be dangerous"), there is a deeper, more important issue. Those supplements might be driving down PSA levels.

So what, good deal, right? Well, yes, and, not totally. Some herbs, such as saw palmetto, may be suppressing the PSA levels in your blood—but not necessarily reducing cancer cells. Honesty—oh, Dad and Mom were right—is the best policy.

Dr. Gerald Chodak, a University of Chicago urologist and co-author of the study, said physicians need to be more attentive as well to the popularity of herb and other dietary supplements. "The question doctors should ask their patients should not be, "Are you taking any drugs?" because many men do not regard supplements as drugs," explains Chodak. "The question that should be asked is: "Are you taking any drugs, and are you taking any vitamins, herbs or supplements?"

A 2005 study published in *Integrative Cancer Studies* provides a bit more insight about how men approach complementary therapies during prostate cancer diagnoses and treatments. While women with breast cancer employed integrative medicine to avoid risk of recurrence, be more central to recovery, help manage stress, be more holistic and boost the immune system, guys with prostate cancer went to complementary therapies to "have more control of their recovery." Hmm, seems like those women have some good ideas in there.

GOOD BETS: SUPPLEMENTING SURVIVORSHIP

There is a (dizzyingly) wide spectrum of dietary supplement choices for men with a prostate cancer diagnosis. And yet there's rarely (say it again, "rarely") 100 percent agreement when it comes to vitamins, minerals, and nutrients and how best to battle recurrence. One responsible, helpful way to consider them is in order of potential value, according to what the experts have found:

Selenium: Since the 1980s, studies have pointed to this substance as a prostate cancer inhibitor. The recommended preventive dose is 200 micrograms per day in the form of brewer's yeast (the Center for Science in the Public Interest recommends SelenoExcell high-selenium be listed on the ingredients label). Some recent lab studies are showing that selenium might also be agent to stop cancer cell growth, making it a good idea for most any man, diagnosis or not.

Vitamin D: Surprise, this old-fashioned vitamin is high on the list. Lab and animal studies consistently indicate that D inhibits the growth of prostate cancer cells. But there is a important twist. The form of vitamin D that proves anti-cancerous is called "1, 25 dihydroxy." University of Maryland researchers suggest eating several daily servings of fruit stimulates this form of D, and also that you need to avoid dairy products because they might inhibit this form of vitamin D. Studies are still needed for the dairy qualifier. Another way the body manufactures D is through sunlight exposure (figure 10 to 15 minutes without sunscreen, that's enough).

Modified citris pectin: Impressive animal studies suggest this supplement could be a major player in fighting off growth of galectin-3 molecules, which are present in a wide number of cancers, including prostate. In small experiments, researchers have found both tumor shrinkage and fast-occurring decreases in PSA levels among human subjects; they estimate that it slows a man's personal cancer growth rate by more than 50 percent, on average.

The pectin acts as an anti-adhesive for cancer cells and is not hard on the immune system. One note: This pectin supplement is expensive at about $100 for a month's supply, and it's probably a long way from being covered by insurers.

Dr. Davis Lamson, a naturopathic physician with a suburban Seattle practice and a prostate cancer researcher at Bastyr University, says modified citrus pectin has a solid track record. He cited one study in which patients took doses of pectin before upcoming prostate surgery. Ultrasound images showed significant tumor shrinkage.

Pygeum: This evergreen tree found in central and southern Africa is more widely used in other countries, primarily for treating men with benign enlarged prostates. Lab studies show pygeum extracts might cross over to block the production of cancer cells in the prostate. More research is needed, and be sure to take pygeum only under the care of an experienced practitioner.

Melatonin: Known more for its sleep inducement, this hormonal supplement has been linked to longer survival in men with prostate cancer. One small study reported it improved survival in 9 of 14 men with metastatic prostate cancer. Lab tests indicate melatonin discourages prostate cancer cell growth in test tubes.

Some facts to consider. Melatonin levels are lower in men with prostate cancer than those without cancer. Prostate cancer patients also tend to have lower than normal nighttime levels of this hormone. Plus, each of us will react differently to the standard dose of store-bought melatonin tablets. If taking a whole pill causes morning grogginess, try a half or even a quarter, always working with a qualified practitioner to see if the supplementation is making any difference in your body's melatonin levels.

THE OLD SAW... THE PREVENT DEFENSE

Some supplements are more proven to help prevent prostate cancer or decrease risk, rather than be an active agent during treatment:

Saw palmetto: You might be wondering why this highly-publicized herbal supplement for prostate cancer didn't make the above list. Simple. It is mostly associated with easing symptoms of benign enlarged prostate glands and not as a fighter agent against cancer cells. That said, saw palmetto is the nation's third highest selling herbal supplement, trailing only garlic and echinacea. A good amount of research suggests it works as effectively as the drug finasteride (Proscar) in reducing an enlarged prostate and its related symptoms. But a 2006 study performed at the San Francisco Veterans Administration Medical Center contradicted this scientific wisdom, showing little difference between a saw palmetto supplement and placebo over one year's time.

Mark Blumenthal, founder of the Austin, Texas-based American Botanical Council and a long-time herbal researcher, said that the men's prostate symptoms (moderate to severe) might have skewed the study's finding. "I don't fault them for raising the bar," says Blumenthal. "I do think it's unfortunate they didn't raise the dosage (from 160 milligrams twice daily)." Proof enough for us: Blumenthal has been taking saw palmetto for about a decade.

Vitamin E: There is a fair amount of research to suggest that a daily vitamin E supplement can help protect your prostate from cancer. The recent wrinkle is that a certain form of the vitamin, gamma-tocopherol, is the most efficient protector.

Zinc: Oregon State University researcher Emily Ho reports that the Government's recommended daily intake for this mineral is 11 milligrams for men and 8 milligrams for women, and that 70 percent of Americans don't get that much. That's a formula for zinc supplementation, which, as it turns out, can have a protective effect in men.

"The link between zinc deficiency and cancer has now been established by human, animal and cell culture studies," says Ho, who is on staff at OSU's Linus Pauling Institute. "We also know that zinc status is compromised in cancer patients compared to healthy people." Even so, Ho warns against taking too much zinc. She cites studies showing men who take megadoses (100 milligrams daily) or use it longer than 10 years can increase their cancer risk. The U.S. Institute of Medicine has established 40 milligrams as an upper limit, but Ho recommends 15 to 30 milligrams as a more sensible dose for men.

ON THE RADAR

Several herbs and botanical medicines have shown some promise for fighting prostate cancer cells, including red clover, African wild potato, pumpkin, rye grass, African plum and stinging nettle.Studies are limited, and none of these herbs have reached any sort of critical-mass status with even holistic practitioners, but it seems to be safe to take them in small to moderate doses: Use this one with caution: rauwolfia. It is a potent herb used currently by naturopaths for blood pressure management.

PC-SPES SLIP-UP

During the early part of this decade, the supplement PC-SPES was winning all sorts of fans among prostate cancer patients and some practitioners. A big reason was the supplement seemed to drive down PSA levels in a hurry. Plus, it was working to extend the lives of patients with advanced prostate cancer.

By 2004, however, the roof had caved in on PC-SPES's foundation, which had been built on anecdotal reports, not rigorous scientific study. Researchers from California and the Czech Republic discovered the product (manufactured in China and distributed in the U.S. by a single firm) contained some powerful synthetic drugs, including the synthetic estrogen diethylstilbestrol, the potent anti-inflammatory drug indomethacin and the popular blood thinner warfarin. Those results, reported at the April 2004 meeting of the American Association for Cancer Research, led the government to demand PC-SPES be pulled from the market.

The PC-SPES formula also included a host of herbs that appear to be worthy of further study: reishi, baikal skullcap, rabdosia, dyers woad, mum, San-Qi ginseng, Chinese licorice and saw palmetto. During the years the product was on market, doctors had suspected that the combination of herbs was causing estrogen-like side effects, such as tender breasts and breast enlargement in male patients. When the ingredient research was presented, physicians realized that the diethylstilbestrol (known as DES) was causing those side effects. Other troubling side effects included blood clots (also possible with estrogen therapy) and excessive bleeding (one Seattle man was found to have warfarin in his blood workup despite never having taken the drug).

PC-SPES doesn't appear headed back to the U.S. Yet some physicians have adopted DES as a still-suitable therapy for men with advanced prostate cancer. The difference is they now are aware of the potential problems and can control the dosage to maximize treatment and limit side effects.

THE Z-FACTOR

There is considerable buzz among prostate cancer practitioners about the herbal product Zyflamend, an olive-oil based extract. Columbia University researchers have shown that it can suppress prostate cancer growth and induce prostate cancer cells to self-destruct. Chief investigator Dr. Debra Bemis calls it a "chemopreventive" effect. She and Dr. Aaron Katz, director of the Center for Holistic Urology at Columbia, have been involved in testing the extract for several years. They have observed Zyflamend significantly decreasing inflammatory COX-1 and COX-2 enzyme activity, which appears to be related to prostate cancer growth.

"We believe one of the main causes of prostate cancer is early inflammation of the prostate, known as prostatitis," says Dr. Katz. "What we are trying to do is reduce inflammation, perhaps through natural or herbal approaches, and thereby reduce cancer incidence. "Dr. Katz pointed out that Zyflamend efficiently disrupts the COX-2 enzyme in a fashion similar to the drug Vioxx, but without the side effects. Vioxx was banned from U.S. sales because it caused serious heart problems in some patients. Zyflamend, available from the New Chapter company, contains a proprietary formula of holy basil, turmeric, ginger, green tea, rosemary, hu zhang, Chinese goldthread and barberry, oregano and scutellaria. Leading natural health physician and author Dr. Andrew Weil has talked it up in print, especially because it gives you a potent daily dose of ginger and turmeric, which he says can be used in cooking, "but it would mean consuming a lot of both herbs on a daily basis."

BEYOND HERBS

When men turn to holistic therapies beyond herbs they usually do so to ease the side effects of diagnosis and treatment, plus improve their quality of life. For instance, acupuncture can neutralize nausea and hold down the vomiting associated with certain types of chemotherapy. Acupuncture is also effective in reducing pain and is officially recognized by federal health authorities for this action. Research suggests that massage therapy can decrease stress levels (always a good idea when fighting disease or protecting against recurrence). It no doubt can improve your quality of life if fitted into your week's or month's routine.

Perhaps the most directly valuable holistic therapy beyond herbs is biofeedback. New research, including a 2006 University of Alabama-Birmingham study published in the mainstream *Journal of Urology*, shows that preoperative biofeedback helped men better learn and perform the pelvic floor exercises (Kegels) that are so vital to regaining continence after surgery.

In the 2006 study, the biofeedback involved using a probe that measured abdominal pressure and external sphincter contraction. The instant feedback was used to better instruct the patient how to contract the sphincter muscle while keeping the abs relaxed, the ideal situation for bladder control. Six months after surgery, 20 percent of men in the control group (who were taught the Kegels with no biofeedback) reported severe incontinence, compared to 6 percent of the men who learned with biofeedback as part of the training. For an issue so important to men undergoing surgery, that's a noteworthy difference.

CHAPTER 7

Health Insurance, Job Solutions

Bob Condor, Curtis Pesmen

Moving into the late 2000s, it's safe to say, health insurance has never been trickier—especially for cancer survivors. At the same time, choices for treatment and control of prostate cancer have never been more varied. So without slipping into the maw of Medicare's reimbursement politics (just yet), the near-term view for survivors and their financial paths offers a few real-world solutions:

First, men employed by an established company and/or insured through a group plan have a good chance of uninterrupted, well-covered, prostate treatment and survivorship care. Job security, as we'll see below, is paramount. (One leading light: the National Coalition for Cancer Survivorship (NCCS) (301) 650-9127 www.canceradvocacy.org)

"One of [every] five cancer survivors younger than 65 delays getting necessary care, or may not receive such care at all, due to cost...."

—Reuters news agency, 2006

111

Second, survivors who are no longer employed and too young to qualify for Medicare benefits, have fewer, but still helpful, accessible options. (One leading source: Patient Advocate Foundation (800) 532-5274 www.patientadvocate.org)

Third, survivors who are covered by Medicare may find bumps in the road—and some severe potholes—in trying to navigate their ways through treatment. Especially if they face a recurrence or find themselves on long-term, preventive, control-the-PSA drug treatment. But here, too, there are ways, as we'll see, to smooth the way or prepare for the bumps. (One helpful solution: Needy Meds (215) 625-9609 www.needymeds.com) The Needymeds.com web site averages 6,500 visitors a day and will soon record its 7 millionth visitor. The site identifies over 350 different companies/programs offering more than 2,600 different drugs and dosages and describes nearly 200 state programs that help with the cost of medicine.

ACHOO! COWORKERS (THINK THEY MAY) CATCH YOUR CANCER

Back in 1996, Amgen, the California-based biotech firm, commissioned a survey of 500 (employed) cancer survivors, 100 supervisors and 100 co-workers of cancer survivors. The results provide a sobering perspective of on-the-job bias, just a decade ago: While researchers found that 81 percent of the survivors felt their jobs helped maintain emotional stability during cancer diagnosis and treatment, the survey also showed supervisors were likely to overstate a survivor/worker's lost time and productivity. For instance: 85 percent of supervisors said fatigue was a major side effect suffered by cancer survivors on the job, while 58 percent of the survivors cited the problem. Three-quarters of the supervisors said they thought the survivors experienced potentially life-threatening infection, fever or low white blood cell counts; but only 41 percent actually reported such side effects.

Donna Doneski, a communications manager at the National Coalition for Cancer Survivorship in Silver Spring, Maryland, remembers a business magazine survey during the same time frame that revealed a surprisingly large number of respondents who still considered cancer to be contagious.

"I mean, 'No, you can't catch it,'" says Doneski. "People with cancer are more outspoken today on the subject of leading normal lives. That's progress, but getting health insurance or your job back still depends on who you are, where you are and what your job is."

BACK TO WORK, BACK TO PLAYING, BACK TO PAYING...THE BILLS

"The biggest role the Americans with Disabilities Act (ADA) plays for cancer survivors going back to work is it discourages discrimination in the first place," says Barbara Hoffman, general counsel, National Coalition for Cancer Survivorship. Not unlike most cancer activists, Hoffman got involved because a loved one suffered through the disease—herself. As a 19-year-old, she was diagnosed with Hodgkin's disease. She clung to her goal of becoming a lawyer, vowing at an idealistic age to help people with illness and disability. Her adversity was our gain. These days, Hoffman is one of America's leading authorities and activists on the employment rights of cancer survivors.

In a few key ways, cancer survivors' quality-of-life has improved on the job and in health insurance circles since the ADA became law in the early 1990s. (Not nearly as much as Hoffman and many of us would like, mind you, but it's gotten better.) One main reason is employers are more aware that people diagnosed with cancer do return to productive careers in the workforce. Another factor: Size. Roughly five of the 10 million cancer survivors in the U.S. today plan to return to jobs and careers (or in the case of childhood cancers, start them). We are far less likely than a generation ago to be denied the normal job and health insurance parts of the very normal lives all cancer survivors desire.

THAT'S THE GOOD NEWS...

"We have successfully persuaded most everyone to use the word 'survivor' instead of 'victim,' " says Hoffman, also a law professor at Rutgers University in New Jersey. "The ADA has helped changed those perceptions." Laws have a way of doing that. So does that fact that virtually everyone knows a friend or family member who has overcome cancer. We see examples of normal, productive lives led by cancer survivors every day.

But, and there's always a "but" when you're talking jobs or insurance, cases such as these "overheard" on the National Cancer Institute's (NCI) colorectal cancer chat lines(www.cancer.gov) are still more here-and-now than anyone would want to admit. "After I had my colostomy, my employer asked me to quit my job because the cancer was upsetting my fellow workers," said survivor/patient Jon H. "He said a demotion or transfer was possible if I didn't agree. Except for my wife, that job was my whole world. So rather than quit, I decided to fight for it."

In a slightly different vein, survivor Roy P., recalls, "When I went back to work, my boss was honest with me. She said that my situation had been discussed at a managers' meeting. Some people had questioned what impact my coming back would have on the company's insurance rates. Her boss asked how she planned to get the job done with an employee (me) she could no longer 'count on' to stay healthy. Fortunately, she did some research and found out that the turnover rate, absenteeism records and work performance of people with a cancer history are very much the same as unaffected workers. Her facts helped correct management's wrong ideas."

When a survivor has been wronged by a health insurance carrier or employer, one area in which the ADA falls short is in effecting a clear remedy.

"Lawsuits don't always get the results you want and they cost money," says Hoffman. These are two solid reasons why any cancer survivor needs to be proactive about the vital issues of health insurance and job rights.

NEW COSTS OF CANCER CONTROL (PLAN D)

Fact is, In January, 2006, the new Medicare Part D program went into effect—a public/private program which is supposed to help provide prescription drug coverage for Americans. Fact is, in late 2006 and into 2007, patients, doctors and pharmacies are still wrangling with key problems of the super-sized federally-backed insurance plan. Not long ago, in a detailed report, *The New York Times* stated bluntly, "thousands of people who take pills to fight cancer have suddenly found themselves with new bills to pay for their essential medicines."

Fact still is, every Medicare recipient, regardless of income, is eligible for the recently expanded Part D prescription drug coverage, Plan D. Yet many patients who had their cancer drugs formerly covered by Medicare, charitable foundations or by the drug makers themselves, must now pay $3,600 per year in new co-payments. The health insurance trade calls it the "doughnut hole," meaning you've got to "get through it" to get to the "good stuff," the full reimbursement. For too many, patients say, the $3,600, or a hefty portion of that, is a whopping, untenable bite.

While it presents a dizzying array of plans and rules, Medicare advises individuals to regard cost, convenience and coverage when choosing their Plan D coverage. Know what you are taking and the cost. Experts also advise patients to create a list of all medications they are taking and why. This would include generic and brand names, therapeutic class, dose, number of pills per month and current cost. Discuss with your physician(s) your choices within a therapeutic class, and possibly switching to a less expensive or generic brand name drug.

Save all paperwork during this period, insurance pros also advise. Steven Hahn, a spokesman for AARP, the membership and lobbying group for older Americans, has gone on record saying that once patients work through the upfront co-payments, Part D provides excellent coverage for cancer drugs. But the high initial cost can be frightening, he conceded.

UNSEEN COSTS OF PROSTATE (AND OTHER) CANCERS

Not long ago, one of the co-authors of this book, a cancer survivor, opened a bill from a hospital where he'd had a CT scan, and was surprised to find the "cost" of this X-ray, a chest-abdomen-pelvis CT scan, according to the figures in the "charges" UCSF column, was $7,818.00.

That's a heavy hit for a 20-minute automated X-ray of sorts, plus a follow-up study. And these days, the near $8,000 procedure may not even produce a piece of take-home film for the patient: The pictures may remain forever stashed on a hard drive or computer server as a series of coded ones and zeroes. Fortunately in this case, the co-author, Curt Pesmen, had reasonable, PPO health insurance when he submitted to the CT exam, so he ended up paying just under $1,000.00 out-of-pocket for his scan. (Even more fortunately, he told me later, the results came back "N.E.D.," for No Evidence of Disease.)

But this relatively simple scan raises lots of questions for survivors—of prostate, breast or colorectal cancer (the kind Curt had). When costs, at some point, become burdensome or prohibitive for follow-up care, at what point do patients begin to delay or forego care their doctors have suggested they have, for proper surveillance? At the $2,000 mark? Or $5,000? What about when new biological therapy (newer than chemotherapy) costs in excess of $40,000 per year, as some new drugs surely do?

GETTING YOUR JOB BACK, OR A NEW ONE (PART I)

In total, 40 percent of people diagnosed with cancer are adults in the work force. They want to go back to their jobs and careers after treatment. Four out of five indeed do return to work, while research shows cancer survivors are no less productive or absent from work than other co-workers.

Straightforward talk with your employer, especially your supervisors and key co-workers, is the best way to disarm any notion that you can't return to the workforce or the job you held before treatment. One point to make clear is the treatment period is naturally going to be more challenging than the months and years that follow once you've put cancer behind you.

The federal Family and Medical Leave Act can be an ally. It requires employers with 50 or more employees to provide up to 12 weeks of unpaid but job-protected leave to address your own serious illness. It also requires employers to continue to provide health insurance and other benefits during the leave period, plus give back your position or its equivalent when you return.

For starters, you may ask, "How do I get health insurance with this now pre-existing condition of cancer? How will employers look at my resume' with the gap of professional experience that matches up with surgery and other treatments? How should I respond to questions about my health?" The National Coalition of Cancer Survivorship or NCCS makes these cogent recommendations for reducing "the chance of discrimination" when seeking a new job:

Do not volunteer that you have or have had cancer unless it directly affects your qualifications for the job. Don't ask about health insurance until after receiving a job offer and only then ask about the "benefits package."

GETTING YOUR JOB BACK, OR A NEW ONE (PART II)

Another key caveat: Do not lie on the job or insurance application. If you are hired and your employer later learns that you lied, you may be fired. Or insurance may refuse to pay benefits and/or cancel coverage. If possible, seek positions with larger employers. Hoffman, for one, believes they are less likely to discriminate or be misinformed than smaller companies.

Keep in mind your legal rights. The ADA stipulates an employer cannot ask about your medical history nor request medical records before making a conditional job offer. If there is a conditional offer, the employer can ask for medical records or an exam only if it is required of all job applicants.

Also, keep the focus on your current ability to do the job. Be confident and avoid sounding defensive. If you have to explain an extended work absence, do it in a way that shows your illness decidedly in the past tense. Hoffman recommends substituting the name of your exact cancer ("lymphoma" or "adenocarcinoma") to avoid using a word that still carries myth and misperception. It is a wise move to have a note from your doctor on medical center stationery to vouch for your ability to perform job duties. Plus, it should reflect your current good/competent health status and the expectation you will likely have normal longevity. The NCI suggests working with a career or jobs counselor to put your best foot—and health outlook—forward.

One oft-overlooked point: "Don't discriminate against yourself by assuming you have a disability," says Hoffman. She urges survivors to make an honest assessment of work-life capabilities—then develop a targeted job search to reflect the assessment.

FROM SURVIVOR TO "INSURED SURVIVOR"

Aside from the formidable physical damage described elsewhere in these pages, cancer wreaks financial havoc as well. For instance, losing a job— or not quite focusing on it while fighting to regain your health—brings the additional collateral damage of jeopardizing your health insurance coverage. Especially if—as with most Americans—you are tied (at least partially) to a group health insurance plan.

Here, cobbled by experts, is a short course on what you need to know about keeping or getting (new) health insurance after cancer. For more tips and details, consult the Resources box for new developments. One other key move: Request the latest revised (that's important) copy of "What

Cancer Survivors Need to Know about Health Insurance" from the National Coalition for Cancer Survivorship (NCCS) and make it your unofficial bible for insurance matters (www.canceradvocacy.org). Karen Pollitz, one of the co-authors of the NCCS booklet, routinely speaks to cancer survivor groups for 45 minutes to an hour. Her most important advice?

"Your protections [to keep or find health insurance] depend on where you live, very much where you live," says Pollitz, project director of the Institute for Health Care Research and Policy at Georgetown University.

PRE-EXISTING CONDITION QUESTIONS

When you first join a group health plan—either after finding a new job or as a cancer survivor (or both)—you'll likely be asked about your medical history. What to do? Or when you make a claim during the first year of coverage, the insurance carrier can check to see if you received drugs or other treatment that would indicate a preexisting condition. If so, the insurance carrier might apply its "preexisting condition exclusion," and deny coverage or reimbursement for up to a year.

Having a preexisting condition, however, such as "prostate cancer two years ago," does not mean you will not be covered. It depends on your plan, as well as the timing. Importantly, a condition is defined as "preexisting" only if diagnosis, medical advice, care or treatment was actually received or recommended during the six-month period ending on the date you enrolled in the group health plan. This means if you're cancer survivor who doesn't require any special follow-up care or monitoring, no preexisting-condition waiting period can (legally) be administered.

Heading out of 2005, five states have decreed all residents be guaranteed individual health insurance, no matter the circumstances: New York, New Jersey, Maine, Vermont and Massachusetts. There are four other states and a capital in which the Blue Cross Blue Shield Association must sell you an individual policy: Michigan, Pennsylvania, Virginia, North Carolina, plus the District of Columbia—Washington, D.C.

LAWS AS HEALTH ALLIES

On a national scale, two laws known as COBRA and HIPAA serve as allies for cancer survivors. They provide protection in many cases, but it is vital to know how and when these laws apply in your individual state. COBRA (Consolidated Omnibus Budget Reconciliation Act) requires employers to offer group medical coverage to employees and dependents whom otherwise would lose group coverage by quitting, getting fired or having their working hours reduced. The national law requires COBRA insurance to be offered by any company with 20 or more employees. Some states have "mini-COBRA" laws that require the same of small companies with less than 20 workers.

COBRA basically "buys" you time to enroll in another health insurance plan, though you have to pay your former employer's part of the premium. You are allowed 18 months of COBRA coverage to make the transition to another health plan.

HIPAA (Health Insurance Portability and Accountability Act), also known as the Kassebaum-Kennedy Act, is intended to help individuals with serious health conditions by removing past barriers (such as turning down a person with preexisting conditions) when trying to get health insurance or keep it when changing jobs. Specifically, HIPAA requires "nondiscrimination" among group health plans

This means group health plans cannot single out cancer survivors because of health status in order to deny, limit or charge more for health coverage. Key fact: In short, if you had an individual plan in place before the cancer diagnosis, it cannot be canceled. Note that this is how HIPAA works for groups. If you need to buy individual health insurance, once again it matters greatly where you live. In some states, insurers can deny coverage, charge higher premiums or refuse to cover any preexisting condition. Other states, as mentioned, have fixed this injustice. But you will still pay higher premiums because it is an individual plan that doesn't afford the economies of scale provided by a larger group. "Beware of any inexpensive health insurance," says Pollitz. "It will be too good to true. Health insurance is expensive."

Pollitz often tells a story about enrolling a fictitious, 46-year-old, breast cancer "survivor" of seven years, in order to test different health plans in Miami and Albany, N.Y. In Miami, out of seven plans, one company turned her down flat (illegal in Florida), one offered limited coverage and five offered policies ranging from about $300 to $1,200 per month. In Albany, the same imaginary enrollee landed offers from all 10 health insurance plans but at much more affordable rates: $200 to $400. In the end, what HIPAA does for individual insurance buyers is... guarantee renewability.

NEW WAYS TO PAY FOR PRICEY PROSTATE Rx'S

By this point, almost goes without saying that even the best, most popular anti-cancer drugs often end up being beyond affordable for everyone. Needy Meds, a nonprofit group started by a doctor in practice, helps with resources all on one website. "Some of the drugs are very expensive and this can pose a real problem." Says Rich Sagall, MD, founder of Needy Meds.

KEEPING YOURSELF COVERED... AND CURRENT

Here's how to aim for—and receive—the best care and coverage from your health insurance provider.

- Keep exact records of all medical expenses. If you are too sick or fatigued, hire a health-claims processing firm [for referrals, try the Claims Assistance Professionals group, at www.claims.org] if you can possibly afford it. It may pay for itself quickly, plus relying on a loved one is a(nother) huge load for that person.
- Send your claims in on time.
- If your claim is denied, appeal it. And appeal it. And appeal it again if you must. One claims-wizened veteran, who's battled insurance companies for years, says working with insurance claims is like a stare-down, or what he calls "a wear-down." He who blinks first or gives up on claims first, loses.

Of special note for cancer patients: Don't settle for an insurance carrier denying use of "experimental" drugs or other treatments. State laws are becoming more progressive to allow consumers access to new treatment options that might be slow to pass federal approval.

For instance, some chemo drugs are officially approved for one type of cancer but routinely and effectively used by physicians to attack other tumors. As a result, insurance companies might try to deny the cost of those drugs. In this case it pays to inform the insurer that you plan to hire an attorney (one experienced in insurance matters). The National Coalition of Cancer Survivorship reports that "courts have generally sided with cancer patients in these circumstances."

"As president of Needy Meds [needymeds.com], I can't speak to the issue of insurance," Dr. Sagall says, "but I can tell you about the pharmaceutical patient assistance programs. These are run by the manufacturers that help those in need who can't afford their medications. Each program has its own guidelines; we check them regularly to make sure our data is current.

"NeedyMeds started when I was discussing PAPs [patient assistance programs] with a medical social worker-friend," Dr. Sagall says. "She had started a database of this information for her own use. One thing led to another, and NeedyMeds was born. Our goal at that time was to provide the information in an easy to access format and without charge. Since then the website has grown considerably. We average over 6,500 visitors each weekday to the website. We have expanded the information we provide and are adding new sources of help all the time."

Then there is always Canada.

BRING IN THE CAPS, NOT THE CPAS

If, comes a time, you are overwhelmed by the complexities of the insurance world, there are professionals who do that for a living. They charge from less than $50 an hour to more than $150 per hour for complex cases and specialize in making sense of incorrect or over-inflated hospital and medical bills. These under-the-radar experts are called Claims Assistance Professionals—CAPs, instead of CPAs—and the members' not-for-profit association, ACAP, has extensive referral lists by state.

One quick tip? Make sure, the CAPs advise, to get all your required authorizations before seeing a specialist for a second or third opinion— and make copies of these authorizations for your records. "It's not easy to prove that you tried to get authorizations," says Susan Dressler, owner of Health Claims Assistance, near Chicago.

ONE SURVIVOR'S Rx STRATEGY

The question to the 6-month survivor, post-radiation, was a simple one: "So how do you pay for your prostate meds?"

"Our biggest problem is the $443 bill for a month's supply of the hormone pills," came the reply from his wife, a patient advocate. "The first day after Jack's first radiation treatment, he stops at our local drug store and buys it. Later we learn that by using a Walgreen Prescription Discount Card, we can get a 10 percent discount. Our Blue Cross Blue Shield Members First discount card gives us another 10 percent discount. That's still a lot of money, so I search the Web and find that www.CanadaPharmacy.com charges only $229 for the same prescription. We order it. Later we learn the Veteran Administration's Health Care system, where Jack, a WWII veteran, is registered, carries a hormone that can be substituted for the one the doctor originally prescribed. The doctor faxes the prescription to Jack's VA doctor, and they send it to us for $21 a prescription.

"We're not out of the woods yet," offers Jack's wife. "Jack completed the radiation treatments, but has a few months left on hormones. He also plans to take PSAs every six months to monitor the prostate. But now we are sleeping without nightmares."

ONE-IN-FIVE, REDUX

Among cancer survivors, 20.9 percent said in a recent article in the medical journal, *Cancer*, that they delayed or missed getting care due to cost or concerns about costs.

ONE LAST QUESTION

Haven't those 20.9 percent already suffered enough?

THE MONEY, HONEY: RESOURCES

National Coalition for Cancer Survivorship (NCCS)
(301) 650-9127; www.canceradvocacy.org
NCCS's promotes awareness of issues affecting cancer survivors. It is a superb clearinghouse with a savvy Web site and national experts second to none.

NeedyMeds.com
(215) 965-9608; www.needymeds.com
According to its founders, the Needymeds.com info site has hosted some 7 million visitors. Why the popularity? Perhaps because its mission is so clearly defined: "Information you need to get your medicine." It's not a pharmacy bank nor traditional charity; merely a hellacioulsy popular—and organized—clearinghouse for patient assistance programs (PAPs) and the like. At last count, the site cited over 350 different programs and firms offering more than 2,600 drugs and dosages. Plus, it describes some 200 state programs that help defray the cost of necessary drugs.

Cancer Information Service
1-800-4-CANCER or 1-800-422-6237
A program of the National Cancer Institute (NCI). Nationwide telephone service for cancer patients and their families and friends. The staff answers questions (in English or Spanish) and send free National Cancer Institute booklets about cancer. They also provide local resources and services. www.nci.gov

1-800-ADA-WORK or 1-800-232-9675
A free service of the President's Committee on Employment of People with Disabilities. It helps employers create accommodations for disabled employees. Offers a wealth of modern guides and wisdom about getting, keeping and maximizing health insurance. Plus, a comprehensive, USA-TODAY-style guide to state insurance departments.

(continued from previous page)

AARP (www.aarp.org)

Has been active in Medicare legislation. Offers a clear, easy to follow website, updated frequently, complete with tools to work out drug costs.

The Plan Finder

http://www.aarp.org/health/medicare/drug_coverage/plan_finder_pdf1.html

Helps with finding Medicare plan that's right for you.

The Medicare Rights Center

Offers a guided tour through its maze. www.medicarerights.org

The government website for Medicare, www.medicare.gov, is loaded with options and information. Be familiar with your current medical coverage and medication needs; the planning tools ask you to punch in this personal information.

Amercian Cancer Society

1-800-ACS-2345

Ask for the free booklet, "Your Job, Insurance and the Law."

Cancer Care, Inc.

1-800-813-HOPE or 1-800-813-4673; www.cancercare.org

Provides free help to cancer patients by offering information on cancer treatments, financial assistance, and other support services.

Health Insurance Association of American (HIAA)

1-202-824-1600; www.hiaa.org/consumer

Its members include the large, sprawling health insurance companies and HMOs that people love to criticize, yet here they're giving back: The association and site provide insurance guides for survivors and consumers on topics such as health insurance costs, managed care, disability income, long-term care, and medical savings accounts.

CHAPTER 8

Putting Cancer in its Place

Curtis Pesmen

For any man who learns his prostate contains cancer, life in the days and years from that day forward will always be viewed through a different lens. Always a cloud in the sky, you could say, even when the prognosis calls for mostly blue skies. Yet, because the overwhelming majority of prostate cancer patients survive longer than the cancer "industry standard" five-year-survival marker, it's tough to say exactly when it's okay to begin to let your guard down—if ever. If you aren't ready to put your cancer "behind you," how, then, do you put it in its place?

"I just had my 10th anniversary," says excited survivor Ron Kauffman, 61, of Jupiter, Florida. "I was 51 when I was diagnosed [PSA of 7.2, Gleason score 6] and had my surgery. I was in a WAR against it. Someone had to win; from my perspective, it really was war." Kauffman is speaking to a five-year cancer survivor—me—by

> " Being diagnosed as having prostate cancer is not likely to transform the average husband into a sensitive, articulate man, eager to discuss his darkest fears...with his wife. "
>
> —Michael Korda, editor, author, *Man to Man*

phone, sounding more like someone who has just gotten engaged to be married. I want to know what's in his Wheaties, or whether he's just naturally animated. (To compare, I felt calm, relieved, even quite pleased on my five-year "cure-anniversary." But I wasn't nearly so amped up.)

It turns out Kauffman is a radio talk-show host. That explains his "rapido" delivery if not his volume. But he's also someone who clearly has done his homework. I first learned of his case while researching my father's prostate cancer, through it-happened-to-me writings Kauffman had done for the University of Pennsylvania's Abramson Cancer Center website (click "support" under "Types of Cancer; Prostate Cancer" at www.OncoLink.com).

"The five-year mark," Kauffman tells me, "was huge for me—HUGE—because I'd read everything I could get my hands on before my surgery. (And I am usually not a wonderful patient.) But I followed every instruction given to me and my wife, Lisa. You hear about the five-year mark; you don't hear about the four-year numbers. You don't hear about the one-or six-and-a-half-year anniversaries. My doc said, after five, 'I am really tempted to use the "C" word with you...but I wont call you "cured" till 10 years [after diagnosis]. At seven years I thought to myself: 'We're getting pretty close here.' And at ten years, it was a little emotional. The doc said: 'I hate to say it' (he was being careful), 'but you're cured.' "

2ND OPINION, 5-YEAR CURE

On a trip to Atlanta not long ago, I decided to fire up the GPS and point my Chevy rental to the national headquarters of the American Cancer Society. I sought the latest, best, prostate survival numbers: clear and simple. With just a bit of explanation from the professionals. Then, I figured, the fears surrounding prostate cancer might be better framed. Here's what I found.

• Welcome to the club: Slightly more than 1.8 million men in the U.S. are survivors of prostate cancer—or more than the population of Phoenix or Philadelphia.

• Approximately one man in six (about 17 percent) will be diagnosed with prostate cancer during his lifetime.

• Approximately one man in 34 (about 3 percent) will die of it.

• Over 90 percent of all prostate cancers are diagnosed while still in local or regional areas: the five-year survival rate for these men is nearly 100 percent.

• Less than 10 percent of prostate cancers, when diagnosed, are found to have spread to distant areas of the body. The five-year relative survival rate for these men is about 34%.*

———

* Source: American Cancer Society, 2006. However, and this is a BIG however, the five- and ten-year survival rates are based on men who were diagnosed and treated as long as 8 to 13 years ago! (10 years of follow-up, plus a few years of analyzing and publishing the data.) So when you figure in today's treatment advances and earlier diagnoses, even these "up-to-date" numbers are less optimistic than those that should apply to men diagnosed today, or in the past few years.

3RD OPINION, 5-YEAR CURE

Q: "When can I consider myself cured of prostate cancer?" asks a hypothetical patient in the book, *100 Questions & Answers About Prostate Cancer*, by Pamela Ellsworth, M.D., John Heaney, M.D., and Cliff Gill.

A: "Prostate cancer, like all cancers, does not 'play by the rules,' " the authors respond. "In the strictest sense, a cancer is...'cured' when there is no evidence of any cancer 10 years after treatment."

PHYSICAL FOLLOW-UP

Between years one and 10, your doctors will want to keep on top of your case, with regular (from three months to annual) office visits, PSAs and digital rectal exams. Sometimes CT scans or X-rays also will be ordered. But the longer you remain stable or free of disease, the less often the "oncs" or urologist-specialists will need to see you. As with any serious disease, though, it's still up to patients to report any unusual symptoms to the doctor between visits.

And yes, you've heard them before, but the symptoms commonly associated with advanced prostate cancer include:

- trouble starting urine flow, or frequent urination

- blood in urine or semen

- pain during urination or ejaculation

- feelings of incomplete emptying after urinating

- bone pain

- impotence

Remember: Many of these symptoms also are caused by BPH, benign prostatic hyperplasia, which is relatively harmless.

Remember, too, as Us TOO national support group leader, local Washington-state counselor, and 17-year-prostate-cancer survivor Jim Kiefert pointed out in Chapter One, measures of PSA can, at times, skyrocket above 1,000 ng/mL and patients will survive. He's seen these guys; talked with them; been amazed by how they seemingly put their cancer in its place. And move on.

GETTING TO... NO MORE LEAKS

Sometimes merely staying on your predicted recovery schedule, when it comes to post-surgery side effects, is enough to help shrink the burden prostate cancer places on patients. Stan Rosenfeld, a survivor and patient advocate from Marin County, California, judged his post-op progress in steps as he re-gained urinary control: The more he had, the less prostate cancer seemed to dog him.

"Yeah, I remember the feeling," he says. "It was: 'Hey, this is great. They didn't lie.' The doc said: 'First you'll be dry at night; then when you're standing.' And I was. 'Then when walking, running, and then playing tennis.' I was seeing it work the way the doc said it would work. At each stage, as I got drier, I said, 'Hey I am on track. I remember being very pleased.'"

OFF THE RADAR

Before diagnosis, "My dad didn't have any symptoms," says Catherine Kapphahn, 37, who in 2002 temporarily left her New York City life behind to accompany her widowed father, Dave, to radiation treatments near his Denver home. His PSA was in the 13-14 range and climbing, Catherine says. And by the time of his first radiation treatments he'd already tried one course of "watchful waiting." In all, Catherine and her father attended 39 external beam radiation sessions over eight weeks. Now that he's 77, and nearly five years older, his five-year check-up date and five-year data bring some new concerns. "Especially recently," says Catherine, "when his numbers [PSA] were going up. He decided to do hormone treatment when they climbed up to 20, and 22.

"The cancer was back; he wasn't 'cured.'" 'Here we go again,' Dave said, 'the third time around....' "He'd read the [books]; he'd asked the doctor all these pertinent questions. He really challenged the doctor this time," Catherine says. And yet he wasn't allowed to put prostate cancer behind him. Least not yet.

MINDFUL FOLLOW-UP

After all that's been thrown at us, one of the toughest challenges for any cancer patient is to move on, to trade in our medical status, to stop being (solely) a patient and start being a former, or part-time, patient. No matter what the pathology reports say about "clear margins" (or not exactly clear), the idea of cancer in our bodies Does Not Leave.

In the best of cases, sure, there may be no more weekly doc visits or phone calls. No monthly "bloods." No more sessions with groins tattooed and bodies positioned just so under the radiation "gun." All good. But by extension there's also a tremendous loss of support once treatment has wound down. What do you do? Now that you're normal again? When will those Sir Dignity briefs be history? When will the erectile nerves "spared" during surgery finally be able do their stuff? You wait a few months, hopefully, then a few more. You do this, and soldier on until maybe the five-year mark, or the 10th, when you're officially, medically "cured," This is a long flippin' time.

At the same time, survivors agree, this transition is not as physically tough as surgery, radiation, seeds or hormone/chemotherapy. And it's not nearly so nerve-stunning painful as those ultrasound-guided biopsy zaps. Still, there's no easy way to say it because there's no easy way to do it: How do you shrink the heavy, mindful space that cancer has introduced in your day-to-day thinking, for weeks or months at a time? The fear was—and is—so real. Mortality made itself known, ahead of schedule, in your life, in your house. (Survivors know this stat too well, too: about 27,000 people die of prostate cancer in the U.S. each year, a number that easily exceeds maximum capacity of New York's Madison Square Garden).

4TH OPINION, FIVE-YEAR CURE

"Once you figure out you're going to live, you have to decide how to, and that's not an uncomplicated matter," says Tour de France cycling champ and cancer survivor advocate Lance Armstrong, in his book, *Every Second Counts*. "You ask yourself: 'Now that I know I'm not going to die...what's the highest and best use of my self?'"

5TH OPINION, FIVE-YEAR CURE

In a similar vein, Jeremy Geffen, M.D., a free-thinking oncologist who happens to live in my hometown of Boulder, Colorado, believes one of the most important questions cancer patients should ask has little to do with five or even 10 years from now. "What about next year?" he'll ask his patients, as part of a life assessment program he advocates and practices.

It's not meant to frighten them at all. Nearly the opposite. Dr. Geffen doesn't want survivors to give too much weight, day-to-day, to their disease for too long. So he'll ask—fairly demand—his patients to make a list: "My top 20 goals for next year are..."

In my case, three of those 20 that hover near the top have to do with personal, not professional goals:

• Spend more intimate time (meals, even) with my wife and family

• Designate one day each week to father/son fun

• Connect more fully with people both close to me and (with some who are more) distant.

Among his own cases, many of which he cites in *The Journey Through Cancer*, Geffen finds survivors mention such goals as:

• Stop looking like a cancer patient

• Be less selfish and introverted

• Support my wife and see her through this period of hardship

• Play golf again

This isn't merely wish-list-making, Geffen reminds us. It's a key psychological accounting. Within reason, we needn't wait five years to live better, to live more fully. Could it be he's also reminding us who's in charge here?

MINDFUL HELP, OFTEN FREE OF CHARGE

So when it comes to handling still-haunting fears, it turns out there's a huge difference between putting cancer behind you and putting cancer "in its place." And countless numbers of my fellow survivors agree: We will never completely put it behind us. We can, however, with some time and help, place it in a reasonably ordered space. (I'll never forget the oncology nurse who once told me, early in treatment maybe a month too soon, "You're gonna' have to deal with the bogey man in the closet for the rest of your life. The trick is to figure out how wide you're gonna' decide to leave the door open each day.")

Too many survivors, as I found after a nine-month colorectal treatment and surgery regimen, view managing their post-cancer emotions as another burden. If you acknowledge you still have daily, weekly, whatever thoughts about recurrence, you're being honest, yes. But at the same time you're then succumbing to certain fears. And nobody wants to think of themselves as "weak" at a time when they are expected, rather suddenly and by so many others, to Be Strong.

Here are three places to turn, where you'll be able to tap into other survivors' views of dealing with, or defeating, those stubborn fears of recurrence.

· American Cancer Society (ACS), Man-to-Man program
(800) ACS-2345, www.cancer.org

· Us TOO International, prostate cancer support
(800) 808-7866, www.ustoo.org

· CancerCare professional support services
(800) 813-HOPE (4673), www.CancerCare.org

TALK A LOT, OR A LITTLE

For the rest of us, especially men, talking about blood in our urine, or loss of libido, tumescence or erectile function, or even an occasional loss of bowel control after treatment doesn't come so easily. This may be one more reason why men are especially at risk for advanced disease; not a biological disadvantage as much as a cultural one. We delay doctor visits. And when we do see the doc, we won't always fess up to all the "little" things that don't seem so awful important.

"He got to a point where he wouldn't leave the house," one wife and care-giver tells me, almost incredulously. "After radiation, he had digestive troubles, and didn't feel comfortable going out most of the time." Nor would he, she says, have reported this sudden post-radiation diarrhea to his doctor, without her prodding. Part pride; part embarrassment; part sto-icism borne of a pre-World War II era. It's all of that, and more.

By contrast, women of middle-age or older have had decades of experi-ence in talking with doctors annually about blood, menstrual blood, vagi-nal discharge, sexual or urinary infections. Plus: they've asked how hor-mones and other bodily changes affect their menses (and emotions). This is still New Stuff for the male of the species, even if and when we're led to the exam table by a supportive wife or partner who understands...and who may powerfully affect our lives and recovery.

NO THANKS, DON'T WANNA' TALK ABOUT IT

Terry Real, of Cambridge, Massachusetts, does very much want to talk about it. In fact, Real (also known as Terrence Real, founder of The Relational Recovery Institute near Boston), author of a best-selling book about mood and the male mind, pulls few punches. I interviewed him in person and was glad I made the trip: His empathetic thinking, and low-key demeanor, I'm sure, helps him connect with many men who otherwise mightn't open up. His book, *I Don't Want to Talk About It*, explains in clear language why most men suffer key (and overlooked) emotional injuries that can lead to foul moods and depression, even absent a severe diagnosis like cancer.

"Most men understand the wisdom of relationship, of sacrifice to larger goals, in relation to their career," Real writes. "But it takes some effort to transpose this same wisdom to the care of their own families, their marriages, their friendships, and even their own health." Notice that Real saves "even their own health" for last. He's surprised, even after counseling men for over two decades, that we do not want to believe we have to make true sacrifices for the sake of our own health. (Until, sometimes, it's awful late in the game.) But for work, for career? No problem. Now it seems, post-treatment, we may have some other work to do.

THE PERSON YOU WERE BEFORE

"I am a social worker. I believe in the power of talking," says Diane Blum, executive director of CancerCare support services in New York City, a national nonprofit group that aids survivors with financial and psychosocial problems related to cancer diagnoses.

"Most people will tell you they want to be the person they were before,"

Blum says, "but the survivorship aspect [of cancer] always takes longer than people tell you it will. The more we can send a helping intervention, with our oncology social workers, we can help normalize the process." It almost makes sense, as frustrating as it may sound: Such a slow growing cancer tends to have lingering effects, even long after it's been removed, or radiated/dissipated, from the body.

ANNIVERSARY REACTION

"I can tell you," Ron Kauffman, 61, of Jupiter, Florida, tells me, "that after the first year anniversary [post-diagnosis] you feel so good you've made it. But by 10 years, you almost forget you could have died."

SURVIVOR'S GUILT

Then, too, there is still more we (of both genders) don't talk about: After a war, a holocaust, a plane crash, you often hear people talk about "survivors' guilt." It's a known, studied phenomenon in psychology and psychiatry. Some years ago, I interviewed a Denver sales executive who quietly (for a sales guy, that is) had made a few million dollars in telemarketing and consulting. But instead of hanging all manner of corporate plaques hailing his accomplishments on his office walls, he had hung prominently, alongside his desk, a fading newspaper article that reported on a major, 1991 airplane crash in which 180 people had perished in the Midwest. This man, a cancer survivor, was supposed to be on that plane. He had arrived at the airport so early, however, that he had qualified for a standby seat on a flight that left just one hour earlier…. Survivor's Guilt, perhaps? After all these years? Or does he continue to hang the harrowing clipping as simply a memento to being in the right place at the right time? He likes to think of this event, this near-death experience, as having more than a little to do with faith. The same goes for countless other cancer patients, I've found since my own diagnosis a few years ago. Sometimes, whether we are ready or not, we're forced to "honor" the threats that have so impacted our lives. And ask the larger questions, about life.

Having acknowledged this, though, the reason I still don't talk much about this possible guilt is that I still feel too hungry to survive. And from where I sit, despite mine and all the "NED" (No Evidence of Disease) anniversaries of my cancer brethren, I still believe I'm on shaky ground. I feel true empathy for my fellow cancer patients past and present, but the guilt, from a personal standpoint, I can't yet fathom. Most things considered, the aversion to "celebrating" my survival-to-date probably has to do with a lingering sense of fear, instead of finality. Could it be possible, I wonder, that I won't be totally healed until I feel and acknowledge the haunting, hangdog emotion of survivor's guilt? It's a stage, then, that I don't especially look forward to achieving.

MY POST-OP RE-ENTRY

In my case, the time after post-op was a bit jittery. As I wrote in my journal after I'd left the hospital worlds: "Two years since diagnosis, and I am cancer free. Don't call myself a survivor... yet; feels too early. Don't call myself a 'warrior,' either. That's for the charity-fund appeal and pink-ribbon ad-campaign writers. But I've taken nine months of treatment ('We're gonna pound you,' my radiation doc said); recovered from life-saving surgery with most of my body intact ('Don't stop cutting till you see the table,' my colorectal surgeon said [in jest]); adopted a child; and I have started hugging my family and friends a bit harder.

"Call me middle-aged guy in remission—make that recovery—because the way I see it, remission means merely temporary absence of disease. Call me healthy, but wary."

HAL P.'S SURVIVOR'S GRIT

"Hearing my PSA report of 0.01 a year and a half after treatment ended was a huge relief," says Hal P., "But to be honest, I expected that. And at 77 I probably have a different view than a younger man would.

"Originally, my PSA and Gleason weren't that high, but after watchful waiting for six months, the PSA began accelerating too fast for comfort. So the doctors and I agreed an aggressive, eight-week radiation regimen with simultaneous hormone shots was my best option. I was too old for surgery. I sailed through that treatment and didn't expect any aftermath.

"But there were after-effects. I believe my immune system was dramatically compromised by the radiation—and that led to a severe bout of pneumonia three months later. Also, I became so weak I fell and broke four ribs and ruptured two spinal discs. I had barely recovered from that when I tripped on a chair and broke a metatarsal bone in my foot. I found out I had severe osteoporosis and one of my doctors suggested was caused by the [anti-androgenic] hormone shots. He hadn't known about my family's history of the disease, and I didn't know that was a side effect. If we had known all that, I would have passed on the hormones."

Even two years after diagnosis, I make a mental note, my dad is still talking about his doctor visits and treatment steps using "we," including my mother as, absolutely, 100 percent part of his team.

"Most of my male friends," my dad adds, "who also are around 80, have had some brush with prostate cancer or are waiting for one. Some stopped taking PSAs because they figure they'll die from one of their other ailments. I'm starting to feel the same way. I really don't think about prostate cancer anymore. I'm just grateful for every day."

Putting Fatigue in its Place

When your family and friends are calling (you know from Caller ID), it's tough, at first, to ignore the ring, to not answer the phone. But when you're recovering from prostate cancer—or the radiation or surgery that's still fighting it—there are times where you know you've got to save up your energy for just an hour or two of activity a day. And, cancer patients know too well, talking on the phone (about your body and disease) constitutes activity. Fatigue, we now know, is no small matter.

And in recent years, medical researchers have found that cancer-related fatigue is more important than they had previously believed. In studies at the H. Lee Moffitt Cancer Center in Tampa, Florida, Dr. Paul Jacobsen and colleagues tried treating fatigue with new substances (EPO, for anemia-like conditions, for instance) and medicines, instead of merely relying on talk therapy... and the passage of time. They were pleasantly and repeatedly surprised.

"Fatigue is exacerbated by depression, emotional distress and stress," says Dr. Jacobsen. "And cancer patients experience high levels of stress and distress, especially during treatment." Patients won't always mention their fatigue because they expect it, or feel they should just accept it—the "cancer" part of healing seems more important to discuss. Remember Dr. Real's "don't wanna talk about it" earlier this chapter? Indeed.

"It's the silent symptom," Dr. Jacobsen suggests, "because patients don't realize they are suffering a symptom." Until now, and possibly for months past the last treatment, patients and caregivers haven't realized how many ways there are available to fight fatigue, and to help put this side effect behind them.

For more info on fatigue and related treatment, contact:
CancerCare(800) 813-HOPE (4673) or: www.CancerCare.org

CHAPTER 9

The Good News Guys: New Treatment Ideas

Curtis Pesmen

In these postmodern times, where "cup of coffee" means 20 different things, cancer survivors no longer expect to have just one or two treatment choices. For primary cancer care and through surveillance, there's a veritable world out there; shouldn't we use it?

Once we hear of new, potential twists on top treatments (see Chapter 3), we also hunger to know what still isn't fully known about knocking out prostate cancer. Survivors want in on the latest "maybes": the strategies, tips or curative paths that command attention while further research plays out in the clinics. In this spirit of moving forward, what follows is a brief, survivor-oriented tour of some of the "Good News" guys and gals who are making, or starting to make, modern—no, postmodern—anticancer prostate news.

"Prostate cancer comes in different flavors. It's not one-size-fits-all medicine."

—Howard Scher, M.D., Memorial Sloan-Kettering Cancer Center, New York City, 2006

HOT LINK—A PROSTATE VIRUS DEBUTS

Striding into the San Francisco Marriott on a late February Friday morning, without real warning I came upon an unexpected buzz in the medical conference press room. Something about a possible "cancer virus" was pushing the assembled media types into "capture" mode....

I'd arrived from Colorado to report on a special, three-day prostate cancer symposium organized by ASCO, the American Society of Clinical Oncology. As TV cameras rolled, Eric A. Klein, M.D., of the Cleveland Clinic Cancer Center, was talking excitedly (for an oncologist, that is) to the media about a new "retrovirus" that seemed to appear in the blood of a substantial number of carefully screened prostate cancer patients. (Screened to check if they had certain genetic characteristics, that is.) Technical stuff, but true. And possibly profound. It was soon time for somebody in this crowd to connect the dots: "Could this point to prostate cancer one day being labeled: an infectious disease?" one reporter asked. And if so, couldn't that make this particular cancer a whole lot less feared?

The answers: possibly; yes. This was the first time—February, 2006—that researchers reported linking such a virus (named XMRV), with prostate cancer development. But Dr. Klein and his colleagues were properly careful. They may have made news, but they did not imply they had found that the retroviruses actually caused the prostate cancer.

Of course, nobody could say much about direct cause and effect just yet. Too early in the investigation. Doc Klein and his colleagues were taking about key, but still first, steps. This reminded me of how HIV/AIDS scientists were both excited and careful at first, in the 1980s, once they found a virus seemingly at fault. It took years before they were able to compose combo cocktails of drugs that could manage the AIDS virus in millions of patients so that it became "merely" life-threatening, or even manageable. But not in-the-next-five-years fatal.

And so the San Francisco XMRV retrovirus debut was enough to capture the assembled crowd because it opened up a new way of thinking about future treatments of prostate cancer. Perhaps someday soon a vaccine could prevent the disease altogether. Ask a hundred oncologists, "Is it better to prevent cancer or cure it?" To be sure, 100 oncologists will answer: Prevention preferred.

After Klein's talk, I asked Howard Scher, M.D., of Memorial Sloan-Kettering Cancer Center, a top medical oncologist in the U.S., whether docs might now start to think about such vaccines for prostate cancer. "There's a difference between therapeutic [treating] and preventive vaccine," he said, implying that we should take a breath or two before getting too excited. A preventive vaccine is the tougher nut to crack. "But what Eric [Klein]'s findings do—and they're important—is look at lesions that have formed and what they can tell us about how prostate cancer is formed." Okay, a couple more links in the chain might be needed. Then may we get excited?

COLD CASES—WHEN CRYOTHERAPY RIVALS RADIATION

It would be easy to say that cryosurgery, or freezing-to-kill cancerous parts of the prostate gland (with long, skinny probes), is "hot." But while viewed as exciting by some prostate docs, the statement may not be fully accurate. Although cryosurgery techniques have been used successfully for decades to treat and kill cancers of the skin, liver and pancreas, this "cryo," as its proponents call it, never has enjoyed the kind of wide acceptance radiation and prostate surgery have received. It's "hot," maybe, compared with its former reputation—and many patients are surprised to find its rate of success in controlling prostate cancer is, today, in line with its rivals.

Still, impotence rates of up to 85 percent among cryotherapy vets have kept many patients from considering this "supercooled" (to -40 degrees Centigrade) attempt at cure. The good news, though, is that a recent study of nearly 600 subjects who chose freezing treatment found that: "Targeted cryoablation [cryosurgery] proved to equal or surpass morbidity rates of external-beam radiation, 3-dimensional conformal radiation, and brachytherapy." So the side effects are shrinking, so to speak, in line with or better than radiation or seeds.

That's high praise, or at least highly useful information for doctors and survivors, who may not have considered cryotherapy before. Its other advantages, according to Fred Lee, M.D., of Crittenton Hospital in Michigan, a pioneer in cryosurgery for prostate patients, include: quicker, relatively contained surgery, and quicker recovery times when compared with radical prostatectomy.

The next hurdle? Convincing insurance companies of its advantages—companies that may balk at reimbursing the $13,000+ fees for the procedure (reported by the University of California-San Diego medical center, as less than half as costly as surgery or radiation). But that's, alas, another story.

NO DRUGS, NO SURGERY, NO RADIATION! NO RECURRENCE?

Call him the doctor who doesn't give up. Call him the heart-health doc who bypassed the bypass. And now, what Dean Ornish, M.D., did for sick hearts he seemingly is doing for diseased prostates. He's making these organs more healthful, without drugs.

Back in the 1980s, when no one seemed to be listening, Dr. Ornish, fresh out of medical school and residency training, had a radical idea: "I'll bet we can reverse heart disease without surgery and without drugs." Instead, he came up with a heart-healthy lifestyle "prescription"—yes, somewhat strict, vegan/vegetarian strict—that could improve blood vessels' and heart health and make millions of people take notice. Cut the fat, up the veggies and exercise, and Do Not Cheat, Ornish proclaimed. (And cut the fat he did: only allowing 10 percent of one's daily calories to come from fatty foods, while many people's diets normally contain 30-to-40 percent fat.)

In swift fashion, collaborating with researchers from University of California-San Francisco (UCSF) and others, he conducted serious studies of his groundbreaking cardiac work and got startling results published. Instead of on the operating table, he fixed sick hearts at the dinner table, in the gym and in support groups. And Ornish found himself, before too long, named: a White House health advisor; one of the "most interesting people of 1996" by *People* magazine; and one of the "50 most influential members of his generation," by *LIFE* magazine.

Naturally, he soon decided to use his natural medicine techniques to fix other powerful organs. And so, to the prostate he turned. In a startling article in the Journal of Urology in 2005, Ornish, Peter R. Carroll, M.D., and colleagues from UCSF and Memorial Sloan-Kettering Cancer Center showed that when nearly 100 prostate cancer patients (93 to be exact) were divided into two groups, the group that followed strict fruit-veg-etable-soy-whole grain diets and exercise plans had markedly lower PSAs after one year. Those in the study who followed a watchful waiting regime but didn't follow Ornish's plan saw their PSAs rise after one year. Plus, not one of the Ornish program group needed follow-up care for their prostate cancers within 12 months, while six patients who didn't follow his plan required follow-up radiation or surgery or other major treatment within the year to control their prostate disease.

In brief, experts say Ornish's experiment was the first study to provide measurable results that changes in lifestyle—without chemo or other drugs—can fight prostate cancer. Or, as good guy Ornish says, "Now we have evidence [these changes] can slow the progression of prostate cancer."

EJACULATION SPECULATION: A PROSTATE CANCER SEMEN TEST

Survivors who wish for something better—and more accurate—than PSA tests soon may have to look no further than an orgasm and their sperm. A new, non-invasive test for prostate (and other) cancer is speeding toward the market before 2009 or 2010, according to principals at New York-based Egenix, Inc. and Proteome Systems of Australia.

Details, of course, plus precise, scientific collection methods, need to be worked out and perfected in the next couple of years. But no snickers here: Research using Human Carcinoma Antigen (HCA) markers with test subjects' semen have shown the new measure to be 100 percent sensitive at detecting prostate cancer. This compares with some reports that put the standard PSA test sensitivity at approximately only 30 percent—which leads to many "false positive" or inconclusive readings.

This also is why so many millions of men have undergone unnecessary or excess needle biopsies in years past. The new semen science is based on glycoproteins, recently discovered to be linked to HCA—and cancer cells. The familiar PSA uses a prostate-specific antigen, or protein, but not a cancer-specific one. The good-guy scientists at Harvard Medical School who first figured this one out can take a bow.

BUILDING BETTER BONES, AFTER DAMAGE IS DONE

This wouldn't be the first time women have taught men something. And as a milestone moment for bones, it won't be the last. Turns out, menopause drugs can help (certain) men. Just ask Christopher Ryan, M.D., an assistant professor at the Oregon Health and Science University Cancer Institute, who has studied bone health of prostate cancer patients on hormone therapy and found there are, indeed, real-world ways to improve bones both during and after treatment.

Doc Ryan and colleagues' main finding: that the drugs and compounds women use during menopause—notably, zoledronic acid (Zometra)— also work on men. Or *in* men whose "male" hormone has been greatly depleted by androgen deprivation efforts to shrink advanced prostate tumors and prevent their recurrence. The prime aim is to prevent hip and spine fractions among those who can ill afford a fall, after weeks or months of hormone treatment. (Another, similar compound in terms of bone activity is alendronate sodium (Fosamax).

After sharing his findings with other doctors at a February, 2006, ASCO annual prostate cancer conference, Dr. Ryan said, "What's new about our study is that it shows starting zoledronic acid later is still effective and can recover bond density that already has been lost." The regimen delivered the drug to patients every three months over the course of a year; results were encouraging: Lost bone density returned. The chances of fractures were reduced. All of which bodes well for our aging bodies, especially those of aging survivors.

WATERMELON MEN: SEEDS OF CHANGE

If it hadn't been written by one of the co-authors of this book, I might not have believed it: Great-tasting watermelon might be able to help control prostate cancer. You mean, we mean: Might we soon think of summer-green striped melons as a kind of "nutri-chemo" to prevent prostate cancer?

Maybe, as long as we use the word "might" (as the research isn't complete). Yet co-author Bob Condor, writing in his "Living Well" column in the *Seattle Post-Intelligencer* not long ago, reported: "Penelope Perkins-Veazie...a nutritionist and food scientist at the U.S. Department of Agriculture in Lane, Oklahoma, [has done research that shows] watermelon is loaded with antioxidants to fortify the body, especially carotenoids that can offset cell damage caused by chemicals and sun."

More to the prostate point, it turns out watermelon is especially high in lycopene (see Chapter 4), which is more typically associated with cooked tomatoes. Lycopene first made Big Nutrition news as a protector against prostate cancer in men.

One of the other recent surprises: Perkins-Veazie tested 15 different lines of mini-watermelons and discovered many of the small, football-sized-types are even more loaded with lycopene than larger melons. She and a colleague have developed a specific test to measure lycopene content. She's also found: Room temperature tends to keep more of the anti-cancer nutrients in the fruit, as opposed to refrigerated melons. Don't forget, however, to spit out the seeds, just as you did when you were 10.

THE "411"—NEW INFORMATION ON INFLAMMATION

It wasn't front page news, but don't be surprised if it does hit the front page soon. There may be a solid link between seemingly innocuous, inflamed body tissues and development of cancer. Not long ago, at a national gathering of oncologists, researchers and pharmaceutical types, the ASCO Daily News ran a story (on page 11, actually) about U.S. and European scientists' advances in understanding how certain inflamed tissues (think esophagus in heartburn; polyps in the colon) evolve over years into tumors or distant metastases.

"We believe what is currently called inflammation is a major part of the host response," said John Smyth, M.D., president of the Federation of European Cancer Societies. And he believes it may well have an impact on whether a primary, or first tumor site, cancer spreads to other organs, or metastasizes. "[It's] the old seed and the soil discussion," he said.

An American doctor, Ray DuBois, M.D., of the Vanderbilt-Ingram Comprehensive Cancer Center in Tennessee, chipped in, "There is a cross talk between pathways of inflammation and proliferation," he said, referring to links between long-term tissue swelling and malignant cells. And so DuBois believes the future of cancer control, including that of the prostate, esophagus and colon, will improve markedly once docs begin to treat both of these processes; not merely a tumor already developed. Put another way, he wants to see anti-cancer cocktails that target both proliferation and—here's that word again—inflammation. Tamping down inflammation, maybe even with over-the-counter pain pill derivatives, may bring many as-yet-undiscovered benefits.

BETTER BRACHYTHERAPY: SMARTER SEEDS EN ROUTE?

Seed therapy, or brachytherapy, isn't as new as you might think. Hard to believe, but the first radioactive seeds received by a cancer patient were implanted in 1967, two years before before U.S. astronauts first hop-danced on the moon. The reason seeds seem so "new" is that prostate cancer patients only began choosing and demanding them in treatment en masse in the 1990s.

In brief, brachytherapy uses ultrasound guidance and tiny (rice-sized) radioactive seeds set inside the prostate gland to kill tumor tissue. Said to be as effective against prostate cancer as external beam radiation, the small seeds deliver powerful doses of radiation inside the prostate, while (hopefully) minimizing damage to urinary, rectal and erectile tissues outside the prostate gland. The most common radioactive seeds in use today are those containing radioactive isotopes Iodine-125 and Palladium-103.

But there's apparently a new kid in town, purportedly offering more treatment power, less risk to the patient's surrounding tissues, and potentially less exposure to radiation, as well. It contains the Cesium-131 radioactive isotope, and is FDA-approved. Of more interest to prostate cancer patients concerned about "excess" radiation is that "131 C" seeds have higher energy, but a lesser radioactive half-life; they stay "active" in the body for only about 10 days, compared with 60 days for Iodine-125 and 17 days for Palladium-103.

"We fully expect our 131 Cs seed to become a leading worldwide treatment therapy for prostate cancer and other malignancies," says Roger Girard, CEO and chairman of IsoRay Medical, based in Richland, Washington. It may be too soon to say whether CEO Girard is being accurate or optimistic: There aren't yet scores of studies to say whether using 131 C seeds lives up to expectations, in terms of cancer control and side effects.

For now, it's encouraging enough to know that there's another choice for survivors, and that, while new, the IsoRay seeds have gained the all-important reimbursement codes from Medicare and Medicaid. The FDA approval came in 2003. Which means, in fact, the shorter-half-life seeds aren't as new as you'd think.

POMEGRANATE PSA POWER

First a disclaimer: As a cancer survivor and medical writer, I'm aware it is quite rare that "One Element = One Cure" for a disease as mysterious and powerful as cancer. That said, I was excited to read recently that: Prostate cancer survivors who drank "one eight ounce glass of pomegranate juice daily" for over 24 months had PSA levels that stayed stable four times longer than patients who didn't actively drink the juice. This news comes from a study at the University of California-Los Angeles (UCLA) Jonsson Cancer Center. Good news, no doubt, as the longer PSA values remain stable (and under 4.0 ng/mL), the better the prognosis for a prostate cancer survivor.

But all this, from something as simple as and sweeter than orange juice?

Researchers here focused on PSA doubling time, because patients who have short doubling times—moving from the 1.5 level, say, to 3.0 fairly quickly— tend to have worse prognoses and outcomes. The scientists at UCLA had reason to smile: The average doubling time for patients' PSAs is about 15 months; those in the pomegranate group recorded a doubling time of 54 months. "I was surprised when I saw such improvement in PSA," says Alan Pantuck, M.D, the study's leader. "We're hoping we may be able to prevent or delay the need for other therapies for many patients."

In a follow-up interview with Dr. Pantuck, I felt bound to point out that pomegranate juice is steeply priced in retail stores, often costing nearly $2.50 or $3.00 for a single bottle. That's about double what we pay for other juices. "In those terms, it is a premium juice product," Dr. Pantuck agrees. (He also points out in his writings that a pomegranate juice company paid for much of the research for the study.) "It is more expensive than orange juice. But it is definitely cheaper than chemotherapy—and hormonal therapy that can run tens of thousands of dollars a year. We don't think we are *curing* prostate cancer, but if we can slow down progression...."

"What excites me," he told me, is: "You could significantly impact the natural history of a cancer by something as simple, and complicated [biochemically], as diet." Okay, it is only one study, only one flippin' *fruit*...but it certainly seemed to do that, at least on a small scale.

CHEMO COCKTAILS, PINPOINTING TREATMENT

As Howard Scher, M.D., of Memorial Sloan-Kettering Cancer Center in New York City once reminded me: In treating prostate cancer, there's no such thing as one-stop shopping. Truth be told, I didn't need reminding. I was concerned about my father, post-radiation, waiting for his next PSA, and I was more curious about Dr. Scher's guesstimates about which treatments might make Big News in the next couple of years. He hardly paused. That's when he suggested a market-basket approach. He was, like any good doc, being careful.

Dr. Scher got me thinking and asking about chemotherapy cocktails, or treatment options that might combine chemotherapy and biological medicine approaches. I wanted my father to have new options, if his disease recurred later with harrowing PSA alarms. What I've learned is: The newer "chemo" drugs aren't the same as the established chemo drugs, in that some don't act like chemotherapy-that-kills-all-cells. The newer drugs aren't always called "chemo," either. These tend to be targeted in approach; they are often called "biologics" to set them apart from older, less-focused, chemo. These bio drugs, like Avastin (or bevacizumab, approved for colon cancer), don't kill all cells around the tumor; they target growth receptors or *parts* of a tumor—the blood supply, for example. This is a big shift from trying one-treatment-at-a-time, or one-chemo-at-a-time, which is how many cancers have been treated for decades. And for prostate cancer survivors, chemotherapy—which often has been saved "for last" in treatment strategies—may, with biotherapy, soon play a bigger role.

"The perception has not caught up to the reality yet," says Tom Kirk, 57, president of Us TOO, the national prostate cancer support group based near Chicago. "Chemotherapy can [now] be used earlier in guys with the disease—and effectively." Many combinations of chemo drugs such as Taxotere (docetaxel) and hormones are now being tested, with high expectations. One example, presented to oncologists in 2006, found that, "In [a] study of 1,006 patients, those who received docetaxel [newer prostate chemo] and prednisone [a steroid hormone] every three weeks had a survival increase of 24 percent...compared with [those] who took mitoxantrone [standard chemo] and prednisone."

Point is, as with colon cancer, once a chemo or biological drug has received FDA-approval for a specific use or time frame—end-stage cancer, for example—doctors over time may begin testing and using the drug, in patients with earlier stages of cancer. This is not so much a chemo "cocktail," but a treatment strategy change that's evolving and becoming more personal.

HAL P.'S COMBO TREATMENT: NEW THOUGHTS

Come to think of it, my father, now in prostate cancer remission for over 18 months, already has a war story or two to tell about combo treatments. Yes, he had external beam radiation for early-stage, Gleason score 6, prostate cancer. No, he didn't need chemotherapy for his type of tumor. But yes, he also endured weeks of neoadjuvant hormone treatment to "starve" or shrink the tumor on one side of his prostate before radiation treatments commenced. And to summarize, his PSA moved, in less than two years, from below 4.0 to 4.8 to 7.1—at the time of treatment—and now, with fingers crossed, below 0.1 ng/mL.

So the numbers are good, even as I see him rise out of his favorite family-room easy chair ever-so-carefully, and painfully, at times.... This is partly due, he says, to the punishment his bones took during the weeks of anti-androgen, hormone therapy nearly two years ago (plus arthritis of the spine). Then too, my dad would admit (without being pressured), the pain is partly due to the fact that he'll soon celebrate birthday No. 78. Gravity and age and loss of joint fluids have taken a toll on his musculoskeletal manhood. So even as the era of targeted therapy for prostate cancer hasn't quite arrived, it's clear that bio- and chemo cocktails are on the near-term horizon. Time enough for many to raise their glasses and offer, "Cheers," for the cocktails to come.

Chapter 10

Resources, Support

Bob Condor, Curtis Pesmen

Actually, you could do better than that: You could look it up, then act on it. The following survivor resources are meant to provide thoughtful options or medically-based means for living stronger, longer. They can also help put you more in control of the body you've got going for you. Some are well-known to doctors, nurses and patients; others are less-publicized but invaluable just the same—to caregivers and those who've faced a tough diagnosis and weren't sure quite where to turn.

> " ...you could look it up. "
>
> —author James Thurber
> (and later, Yogi Berra,
> ex-New York Yankees star
> catcher and manager)

A WORD ABOUT HEALTH WEBSITES

While it's a tough slog to obtain complete, unbiased cancer information from any one Internet site, it is the rare patient who consults just one website. "A few good websites," is the educated survivors' goal. Too many may be daunting. And, as always, it's wise to be wary of those websites that seem to be much more interested in selling something than in truly educating those who've clicked their ways in.

GENERAL PATIENT-FRIENDLY SOURCES

■ Us TOO International
Prostate Cancer Education & Support
5003 Fairview Ave.
Downers Grove, IL 60515
(800) 80-UsTOO (800) 808-7866
www.ustoo.org

Originally formed in answer to "Y-Me," the successful, nonprofit breast cancer support groups, this ever-growing organization lives up to its name by providing both insider medical information and well-structured support groups, usually near your home (and that usually meet monthly). For extra, in-the-know advice, consider joining Us TOO's Prostate Pointers online community. You have to give a nod to a group that names its cryotherapy (frozen prostate treatment) newsgroup, "Iceballs."

■ American Cancer Society (ACS)
Man-to-Man program
2200 Century Pkwy. NE
Atlanta, GA 30345-3154
(404) 315-1123
(800) ACS-2345
www.cancer.org

You've no doubt seen the ubiquitous red, white and blue logo of the American Cancer Society before, but less well-known is the ACS Man-to-Man support program, which starts grass-roots and goes a bit deeper. You sign up via phone or computer or your local ACS chapter, which guides you toward your exact needs: information, newsletters, free decision tools, support groups for patients only or related support groups for patients and wives or partners (called "Side-by-Side"). There's also a valuable, medical-journal based program called NexProfiler, available through the ACS website, prostate cancer section, that matches the latest medical studies to your exact survivorship concerns.

■ **Prostate Cancer Foundation** (PCF)
1250 Fourth Street
Santa Monica, CA 90401
(800) 757-CURE (2873)
www.prostatecancerfoundation.org

A quarter billion dollars. Big bucks for a gland. In total as of presstime, PCF has raised more than $260 million to find better treatments and a cure for recurrent prostate cancer. This makes it the biggest private funding group in the world of prostate cancer research, it humbly reports. But one key is that PCF—founded by survivor (PSA 24 when diagnosed) and Wall Street legend Michael Milken—makes research happen quickly. And it helps publicize this research through conferences, books, newsletters, and national events, including working with Major League Baseball and mega-food store chains. Another key is that PCF puts the word "recurrent" in its mission against cancer. Survivors like to see that. Like Milken, PCF is a player. And an educator.

■ **The Prostate Net**
The Prostate Net, Inc.
P. O. Box 2192
Secaucus, NJ 07096-2192
www.prostate-online.com

More than most cancer sites, The Prostate Net seeks to strengthen community. As in local community, not just the cancer community. This 501(c)3 nonprofit started up in 1998, after its founder, Virgil Simons, emerged from prostate surgery at age 48 a (slightly) changed man. Most recently, in '06, Simons' group engineered a community-based networking plan that has barbershops in urban areas posting and distributing prostate information—and reaching an otherwise elusive, middle-aged and older crowd.

■ **American Society of Clinical Oncology** (ASCO)
1900 Duke St., Suite 200
Alexandria, VA 22314
(703) 299-0150
www.asco.org

A Washington-based, must-know group for any person or family diagnosed with cancer ASCO's membership includes more than 20,000 oncologists and other cancer health-care specialists, and its annual medical meetings make news globally, not just in the U.S. For the latest in peer-reviewed "advances" in anti-cancer discoveries, seek out the annual summary report called, "Clinical Cancer Advances," which covers treatment, prevention and screening. (These reports are also delivered to doctors in their "own" magazine, the *Journal of Clinical Oncology*.)

■ **People Living With Cancer** (PLWC, "an ASCO website")
c/o American Society of Clinical Oncology
1900 Duke St., Suite 200
Alexandria, VA 22314
(703) 299-0150
www.plwc.org

The ASCO staff has spent considerable time and money to make PLWC, a patient-oriented website, both authoritative and survivor-friendly. It cites "oncologist-approved cancer information" as its calling card, and has deep roots in the cancer counseling, social work and therapy communities. Plus, it has great, detailed medical illustrations of prostates and other body parts, suitable for taking to your doctor to make more sense of your diagnosis or prognosis.

■ **American Urological Association** (AUA)

1000 Corporate Boulevard

Linthicum, MD 21090

(866) RING-AUA (866) 746-4282

(410) 689-3700

www.urology-health.org

www.uaunet.org

Need to rule out a handful of other "possibles" before concluding any new symptoms might mean cancer recurrence? AUA has a broader educational mission than prostate cancer-specific groups—following (and leading) developments in both male and female urology—but it also has sufficiently tight ties with the more surgically-minded members of the profession. Those with long-term incontinence problems might benefit most from repeated contacts with the AUA.

■ **American Society for Therapeutic Radiation and Oncology** (ASTRO)

8280 Willow Oaks Corporate Drive, Suite 500

Fairfax, VA

(800) 962-7876

www.rtanswers.org

Radiation treatments aren't nearly as simple as in the 1980s or 1990s. Today's decisions, beside the sort that weigh external beam vs. brachytherapy seeds, include different types of radiation simulation, three-dimensional mapping and "conformal therapy, as well as varying doses and "loads" of string- guided radiation seeds. Radiation also is used more frequently in attempts to pre-treat, or "shrink" tumor tissue before an operation.

■ **National Cancer Institute** (NCI)
NCI Public Inquiries Office
6116 Executive Boulevard
Room 3036A
Bethesda, MD 20892-8322
www.cancer.gov
www.cis.nci.nih.gov/news

NCI is a key federal agency, charged with "eliminating the suffering and death due to cancer." Tall order. On your behalf, it runs the Cancer Information Service (CIS) and shares with patients its Physician Data Query (PDQ) database which contains thousands of peer-reviewed summaries of significant research findings. You can find prostate cancer drug trials, follow results of ongoing research, and, at times, begin to see treatment strategies (or protocols) before they're approved by the FDA.

■ **CancerCare**
275 Seventh Avenue
New York, NY 10001
(212) 712-8400 or
1 (800) 813-HOPE (4673)
www.CancerCare.org

"No one should have to face cancer alone," says this national nonprofit group (formed in 1944), which offers free wide-ranging advice. The range of services is dizzying, but not limited to prostate cancer issues. Support and guidance in English and in Spanish are provided by social workers and online chat groups. Plus, this .org runs regular, doctor-telephone workshops, which are broadcast live but archived for later listening, and offer present solutions for a variety of cancer patients' problems.

■ **Lance Armstrong Foundation**
P.O. Box 161150
Austin, TX 78716-1150
(512) 236-8820
www.livestrong.org

If you've read Armstrong's books, you know he's not shy about talking about his cancerous testicle and what happened to it, during his battle with metastatic cancer that had spread from his testicle to his brain. He survived well, he's said, due to four things beyond chemo (which he also reveres): knowledge, support, motivation and hope. "I want to extend these four gifts to all cancer survivors," he also says. And that, along with having raised well over $30 million for cancer research and survivorship issues, is what his fund is about. It also, generously, sends out notebooks, gratis, for organizing medical records and financial info; it also provides low-cost music downloads and DVDs of interest to all survivors—and their caregivers. A Tour de Force of survivorship help, from the seven-time Tour de France champ.

■ **OncoLink Abramson Cancer Center**
Abramson Cancer Center
of the University of Pennsylvania
3400 Spruce St.
Philadelphia, PA 19104
(215) 662-6065
www.oncolink.com

Oncolink, the website, and Abramson, the cancer center of the University of Pennsylvania, are a first-rate anti-cancer team. Rarely do a website and a staff of medical doctors BOTH rate so highly, according to so many patients—and fellow doctors and nurses. As medical journalists (and as cancer survivors, as is one of this book's co-authors), we find ourselves using Oncolink time and again, without apology. Simply put, we trust it in part because it was one of the first, advanced cancer information websites that had an elite med-school pedigree and a massive consumer following. Still does.

■ **Sex Information Council of the United States** (SIECUS)
130 West 42nd Street, Suite 350
New York, NY 10036
(212) 819-9770

Perhaps an unlikely choice for this listing, at first glance, but a closer look (and personal visits) points to SIECUS's amazingly broad collection of books, journals and other scientifically "intimate" materials. In addition, the council boasts an unusually helpful and discreet library staff, in terms of helping you conduct research—from afar if you don't live in New York—on highly personal, emotional subjects. All inquiries are handled with care and respect, from teenagers curious about the risk of chlamydia or HIV/AIDS related to their first sex act.

■ **American Society for Therapeutic Radiation and Oncology** (ASTRO)
8280 Willow Oaks Corporate Drive, Suite 500
Fairfax, VA 22031
(800) 962-7876
www.rtanswers.org

Radiation treatments aren't nearly as simple as in the 1980s or 1990s. Today's decisions, beside the sort that weigh external beam vs. brachytherapy seeds, include different types of radiation simulation (see Chapter 4), three-dimensional mapping and "conformal therapy," as well as varying doses and "loads" of string guided radiation seeds. Radiation also is used more frequently in attempts to pre-treat, or "shrink" tumor tissue before an operation.

■ **Physicians Committee for Responsible Medicine** (PCRM)
5100 Wisconsin Ave. NW, Suite 400
Washington, DC 20016
(202) 686-2210
www.pcrm.org

This "committee" is more than that: It's a doctor-based group that reports on anti-cancer advances related to food, nutrients and lifestyle behaviors. It also runs "The Cancer Project," an ongoing feature in its magazine, Good Medicine, and on its website, that highlights newsier notes (from medical journals and the like) for survivors. One recent example: "Men who have been treated for prostate cancer are less likely to have a recurrence if they maintain a healthy weight, according to...the journal, Urology."

■ **Patient Advocate Foundation**
700 Thimble Shoals Boulevard, Suite 200
Newport News, VA 23606
(800) 532-5274
www.patientadvocate.org

First comes info, then comes muscle, when you're facing financial or other hardships due to cancer treatment, bills and related care. This foundation is all about adding muscle and helping to plug key holes in our nation's leaky health insurance basket. There are no guarantees, as in life, that the case managers can help your particular case, but they draw from a national network of resources and aren't at all shy about suggesting mediation and other methods to help you worry less. A lot less.

HELP VS. HYPE

MEMORIAL SLOAN-KETTERING CANCER CENTER DATABASE

Known for its world-class oncologists and cancer research, MSKCC, the New York City-based center, offers more extensive information on herbs, botanicals and other complementary treatments than many outsiders might expect from such a medically-scientific bastion. www.mskcc.org/mskcc/html/11570.cfm

QUACKWATCH

A treatment too good to be true? When someone tries to pitch you or your family a "wonderful new..." or a so-called "radical cure," one heads-up way to find out if it's got solid science behind it is to head to "Quackwatch." Designed to separate wheat-from-the-chaff and expose hyped-up possibile "cures," this site doesn't believe in giving non FDA-approved medicines, botanicals or other treatment modalities the benefit of the doubt. It's tough, demanding, when it comes to its reporting. Too tough for some patients' tastes? Maybe it has to be. www.quackwatch.orgf/index.html

The University of Texas, M.D. Anderson's Complementary/Integrative Medicine site, www.mdaanderson.org follows the ever-evolving world of CAM (complementary and alternative medicine) regularly and with authority. Updated often, the site includes FDA Advisories and reports on unexpected interactions between various drugs that survivors (or their docs) may not have experienced before.

Acknowledgements

When Curt Pesmen and co-publisher Chris Sulavik of Tatra Press asked me to be part of this book project, I couldn't accept quickly enough. I share their commitment to "patient-first" reporting and storytelling; I admire their tireless efforts to get this book into the hands of countless men with prostate cancer—and the wives and significant others who love them. It's been an honor to help make those connections through these pages.

My personal thank-yous go out to all the patients, current and ex-, including champion baseball manager Joe Torre and Seattle area resident Bob Fuhr. Both men are representative of the enduring optimism I have discovered in prostate cancer survivors. The fact that both are nice guys who are generous with their time is no accident, I'm guessing, and it is probably a direct reflection on their equally giving wives, Ali Torre and Mary Fuhr. Curt and I owe a lot to these two couples and the many others who were willing to be interviewed for this book.

While patients are paramount in this guide, I'm also appreciative of the wisdom of the numerous doctors and researchers who were happy to talk and, more importantly, share their work. A special nod goes to Gerald Chodak, M.D., professor of surgery at the University of Chicago and director, Midwest Prostate and Urology Health Center, who was instrumental in several reports on prostate cancer I filed in my decade as the health writer and columnist for the *Chicago Tribune*.

Likewise, many thanks go to Dr. Davis Lamson at Bastyr University in Seattle, nutritionist Natalie Ledesma at the University of California-San Francisco, Mark Blumenthal at the Austin, Texas, based American Botanical Council and Barbara Hoffman, a Rutgers University law professor and general counsel for the National Coalition for Cancer

Survivorship near Washington, D.C. All were as practical with their advice as they are brilliant.And, practically speaking, my own brand of enduring optimism flows straight from my wife and best friend, Mary, and our two 9-year-olds, Lana and Arthur. I can't write a single word without them in my heart; and wouldn't want to try.

—Bob Condor

After working with Bob Condor at *Esquire* magazine for a short while in the '80s and after editing his work at *SELF* magazine in the '90s, I was truly looking forward to working with him on this project—despite the fact that it is, at its heart, a book about cancer.

But because of Bob's heart, and his mind, from the start I knew this wouldn't be an "ordinary" book about cancer. Beside the biology, it would be about life, accomplishment, health, fitness, and love. (And, yes, it would be about surgery and radiation and sometimes grueling after-effects as well.) I told Bob early on, we should try to make certain those who read this book remember it as much for the survivors' voices, as for the nuts-and-bolts/catheter-and-nutrition advice they will also find inside.

Great thanks are owed to the men and families whose stories are at home here, for we asked them to take us inside their lives, their recovery and radiation rooms, and inside their (normal) zones of privacy. We did so in hopes of relaying to others exactly how it feels to be a modern prostate cancer survivor.

I am indebted to all the generous doctors, nurses, medical assistants,and patient advocates across the U.S. and Canada who agreed to donate their time, and thoughts, to this project. Among those who deserve special mention: Peter Carroll, M.D., chair of urology, University of California-San Francisco School of Medicine; Mitchell Benson, M.D., chair of urology, Columbia University School of Medicine; Jim Kiefert, survivior and chairman of the board of Us TOO International; Tom Kirk, CEO of Us TOO; Sarah Evans and Katie Lambe of the Prostate Cancer Foundation; Diane Blum, Executive Director of CancerCare, Inc., Steve Kurtzman, M.D., radiation oncologist, El Camino Hospital, Mountain View, CA; Daphne Haas-Kogan, M.D., radiation oncologist, University of California-San Francisco, Mark Lane Welton, M.D., chief, colo-rectal surgery, Stanford University Cancer Center, Alan Venook, M.D., chief, gastrointestinal oncology, University of California-San Francisco; and Allen Cohn, M.D., medical oncologist, Rocky Mountain Cancer Centers, Denver.

Thank you Chris Sulavik, Stephanie Bart-Horvath, and Viki Psihoyos, for helping to shape and fortify the look and feel of these chapters. Thank yous are also owed to Heather Goethe and Todd Bentsen in media relations at the American Society of Clinical Oncology, Alexandria, VA, for their help in granting us much-needed access to ASCO members and their findings.

Closer to home, I reached out to my father and mother, Hal and Sandy Pesmen, in many ways I never had before: including son-to-father, cancer survivor-to-cancer survivor. Their guidance and love, along with that from my sister, Beth Preis, anchor of the Northbrook clan, got us all through some unpredictably tough times.

And closest to home, there aren't enough thanks to offer my amazing wife, Paula, and Joshua and Jesse, for their so many hours of patience and selfless support of the writer in the family. It is survivorship of a very different order; and I cherish it daily.

—Curtis Pesmen

Afterword

So now we've heard. From the doctors—and survivors. The PSA tests that measure proteins in our blood aren't perfect. Don't we know. But they're being revised, re-thought, reconfigured. For the better.

We've also heard that radiation therapy aimed at prostate cancer tumors is becoming at once more powerful, less damaging and more precise. And as this applies to both external beams and (implanted) brachytherapy seeds, it too is getting better.

At the same time, marked advances in cryotherapy, chemotherapy (which used to be considered rarely in prostate cancer—if at all), hormone treatments, gene-based drugs and targeted therapies have opened up the treatment field rapidly and immensely.

So it is with prostatectomy, the radical kind; the bloodiest, seemingly harshest treatment for prostate cancer at the outset, that is softening its edges. It is now being re-shaped in major ways by smaller cuts, minimally-invasive tubular scopes, magnifiers and cutting devices; and also by a $1.5 million surgical robot called daVinci. Less blood, smaller incisions, more precision, fewer side effects, the experts enthuse. All for the better.

"Up to now, robotic surgery has been confined to rare or unusual procedures," reports the University of Chicago medical center. Prostate surgery "could be the first common procedure taken over by this approach."

Even trusty, low-tech "watchful waiting" has acquired a new moniker. Depending on the doc and medical center, it might now be called "active surveillance." Which suggests action; not merely sitting or waiting around till the next PSA. In many cases there's more being done between PSAs to gauge and protect the health of the prostate gland—and its owner (including diet changes and an "anxiety scale" for prostate patients under development at the University of California—San Francisco). For many unsteady-PSA patients, this is a subtle-but-welcome change. For the better.

In their entirety all these changes and treatment improvements (if we're still being honest here), can seem overwhelming. Especially if they're presented or downloaded immediately after diagnosis. As Tom Kirk, president of Us TOO International prostate cancer support group, told the authors of this book—only half in jest: "[For some], it's like trying to take a drink from a fire hose." Progress, then, in small sips...and giant leaps.

Yet no matter the treatment, no matter the techno know-how, we can all agree it's time to put the fire out. And tamp it down for a long, long time. Or forever.

ABOUT THE AUTHORS

CURTIS PESMEN, author of THE COLON CANCER SURVIVORS' GUIDE, HOW A MAN AGES, WHAT SHE WANTS and YOUR FIRST YEAR OF MARRIAGE, and who has written for *Esquire*, *GQ*, *SELF*, *Glamour*, *Redbook* and *Outside* magazines, was diagnosed with advanced colon cancer in 2001. As health/features editor of *SELF* magazine, he helped develop the internationally recognized, pink-ribbon breast cancer awareness campaign. An award-winning, seven-part series of Pesmen's (so far) successful fight against colon cancer was featured in *Esquire* magazine in 2001 and 2003. Most recently, Pesmen has written on cancer issues for publications such as: *Money*, *Glamour* and *CURE*. He lives in Boulder, Colorado, with his wife and two sons.

BOB CONDOR is the *Living Well* columnist for the *Seattle Post-Intelligencer* and editor of *Conscious Choice*. Additionally, he freelances for numerous publications, including *Best Life* and *Life* magazines. Condor is author of MICHAEL JORDAN'S 50 GREATEST GAMES, co-author of MARY LEE'S NATURAL HEALTH & BEAUTY: HEALTHY LIVING WITH ESSENTIAL OILS and A CAREGIVER'S COMPANION.

Previously, Condor was the health and fitness columnist for the *Chicago Tribune* for nearly a decade. He has been nominated for two Pulitzer Prizes, including beat reporting and feature writing, and has won awards from the American Heart Association, Illinois Mental Health Association, National Stuttering Foundation and Chicago Headline Club. Condor also was a writer and editor at the *New York Daily News*. He lives in the Seattle area with his wife and two children.